ENZYME NUTRITION

The Food Enzyme Concept

EAST WEST
807 BLOOR STREET WEST
TORONTO, ONTARIO
M6G 1L8
(416) 530-1571

ST WEST
07 BLOOR STREET WEST
RONTO, ONTARIO
6G 1L8
416) 530-1571

ENZYME NUTRITION

The Food Enzyme Concept

Dr. Edward Howell

With research contribution by
Maynard Murray, M.D.

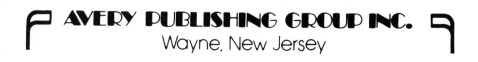
AVERY PUBLISHING GROUP INC.
Wayne, New Jersey

The medical and health procedures in this book are based on the training, personal experience, and research of the author. Because each person and situation is unique, the author and publisher urge the reader to check with a qualified health professional before using any procedure where there is any question as to its appropriateness.

The publisher does not advocate the use of any particular diet and exercise program, but believes the information presented in this book should be available to the public.

Because there is always some risk involved, the author and publisher are not responsible for any adverse effects or consequences resulting from the use of any of the suggestions, preparations, or procedures in this book. Please do not use the book if you are unwilling to assume the risk. Feel free to consult a physician or other qualified health professional. It is a sign of wisdom, not cowardice, to seek a second or third opinion.

Cover art by Tim Peterson
Cover design by Rudy Shur

Library of Congress Cataloging-in-Publication Data

Howell, Edward, 1898—
  Enzyme nutrition.

  Includes index.
  1. Enzymes--Therapeutic use. 2. Nutrition.
I. Murray, Maynard. II. Title. [DNLM: 1. Enzymes.
2. Nutrition. QU 135 H859e]
RM666.E55H68   1985   616.8'54   85—11222
ISBN 0-89529-300-5
ISBN 0-89529-221-1 (pbk.)

Printed in the United States of America

10   9   8   7   6

Contents

Foreword

As a researcher, reporter, and author of over twenty books on nutrition, health, and related subjects, I feel privileged to be able to introduce the concept of food enzymes to you as presented by Dr. Edward Howell in this book. Here is how my own introduction to this excellent work occurred. I read an interview of Dr. Howell on the subject of Food Enzymes in the *Healthview Newsletter*, published in Charlottesville, Virginia. This interview was so impressive, I asked for permission from the editors of the newsletter to write an article about Dr. Howell and enzymes in *Let's LIVE* magazine, of which I am a contributing editor. After receiving permission, I wrote the article for the June 1977 issue of *Let's LIVE*. The response of the public to this information, which stated how enzymes could aid health and prolong life, was so strong that the magazine editors stated that "this article has drawn more comment from the readers than perhaps any article in *Let's LIVE* history." This is due, I am sure, to the helpful potential of the use of enzymes in the daily diet, as explained by Dr. Howell in this book, *Enzyme Nutrition*. More recently, due to many requests of old and newer subscribers who had heard about the enzyme information, this article was repeated in the August 1980 issue of *Let's LIVE*. At the time of the writing of the June 1977 article, the only source of the information appeared in the *Healthview Newsletter* and the *Let's LIVE* magazine. At that time, suggestions were given that Dr. Howell was at work on a complete book on the subject. Many scientists and doctors wrote me asking for information, as well as for the address of Dr. Howell, who had not yet finished the book. This book is now finished, and the full story of how enzymes can help human (as well as animal) health is at last revealed.

This information is a new addition to the history of nutrition and the betterment of health, now available to scientists, doctors, and you, the general public.

Linda Clark, M.A.

Introduction

In the early 1900s, Casimar Funk discovered the vital importance of vitamins in human nutrition and health. Some years later, researchers looked at the then unknown role of minerals and trace elements in health. Again, the nutritional picture took on a new dimension. This book is an attempt to bring into the light the most important nutritional discovery since vitamins, minerals, and trace elements, and perhaps the only solution to our present health crisis—food enzymes. The study of food enzymes in nutrition and human health has been a 'sore eye' to both scientists and nutritionists alike. For enzymes operate on both chemical and biological levels, and science cannot measure or synthesize their biological or life energy.

This biological force is the very core of every enzyme. Various names such as life energy, life force, life principle, vitality, vital force, strength, and nerve energy have been offered to describe this energy. Without the life energy of enzymes we would be nothing more than a pile of lifeless chemical substances—vitamins, minerals, water, and proteins. In both maintaining health and in healing, enzymes and only enzymes do the actual work. They *are* what we call in metabolism, the body's labor force.

Enzyme Nutrition points out that each one of us is given a limited supply of bodily enzyme energy at birth. This supply, like the energy supply in your new battery, has to last a lifetime. The faster you use up your enzyme supply, the shorter your life. A great deal of our enzyme energy is wasted haphazardly throughout life. The habit of cooking our food and eating it processed with chemicals; and the use of alcohol, drugs, and junk food all draw out tremendous quantities of enzymes from our limited supply. Frequent colds and fevers and exposure to extremes of temperature also deplete the supply. A body in such a weakened, enzyme-deficient state is a prime target for cancer, obesity, heart disease, or other degenerative problems. A lifetime of such abuse often ends in the tragedy of death at middle age.

The purpose of this book is to educate scientists, health activists, and lay persons about the enzyme theories that Dr. Howell calls the Food Enzyme Concept. Along with his book *The Status of Food Enzymes in Digestion and Metabolism*, it is the first significant scientific attempt to prove the necessity of raw foods in human nutrition. In it he tells us what enzymes are, how they keep us alive, and the consequences of the present enzyme-deficient diet. In a highly readable and entertaining style, Dr. Howell exposes the crippled attempts of modern medicine to heal disease and its failure to attack the root of the problem. His conclusion is that many, if not all, degenerative diseases that humans suffer and die from are caused by the excessive use of enzyme-deficient cooked and processed foods. With all the billions of dollars spent on university and private research, it seems amazing that the cause of our current health crisis could be so clear-cut and simple. Yet the scientist or lay person who reads this book must respect the conclusions of Dr. Howell and the hundreds of contributing researchers as a significant contribution to the fields of human nutrition, degenerative disease, and aging.

In Chapter 1, the book gives an overview of the Food Enzyme Concept. This is followed by a discussion of the elusive life principle in enzymes and what Dr. Howell refers to as the enzyme bank account or potential. Each of us is given a limited supply of enzyme energy at birth that must last us a lifetime. Key to his theory that man could live longer and be healthier by guarding against loss of his precious enzymes is the example of wild animals in nature, who statistically outlive man and die of only a handful of natural causes. Howell goes on to show that bodily enzyme depletion and aging go hand in hand in both laboratory animals and humans.

Chapter 3 tells us what enzymes are and what they do in our body: they are the workers responsible for every activity of life; even thinking requires enzyme activity. Also in Chapter 3, the enzymes in foods are listed and their use in traditional recipes worldwide is explained in detail. The chapter also shows how animals harness the enzyme power in food by burying or covering it, thus allowing the food enzymes to predigest it, before they return to eat it. In this way they preserve their own precious enzyme supply.

Two important discoveries are discussed in Chapter 4, the food-enzyme stomach and the Law of Adaptive Secretion of Digestive

Enzymes. The latter states that the body calls for exactly the quantity and type of enzymes needed according to the character of each meal eaten. This replaces the false theory of parallel secretion of enzymes which claimed that the organism's three main enzymes, protease, lipase, and amylase, are all secreted in equal amounts regardless of the type of food eaten, raw or cooked. The existence of the food-enzyme stomach in animals and humans is the key to the Food Enzyme Concept. Howell shows that what was formerly called the "idle" cardiac portion of the human stomach is really a non-glandular food-enzyme stomach where sizable quantities of starch and other nutrients are predigested by salivary ptyalin and food enzymes for up to one hour before undergoing the more widely known functions of digestion. The crops of birds, worms, and grasshoppers, the forestomachs of cattle, sheep, and other ruminants, and the huge non-glandular forestomach of the whale are all examples of food-enzyme stomachs in animals.

One fatal process may be the cause of all humanity's bodily ills. If you haven't guessed already, it is the cooking of food, the subject of Chapter 5. Prolonged heat over 118° F kills enzymes; cooking temperatures destroy 100 percent of the enzymes in food. What is left is enzymeless food that makes up the bulk of the modern enzyme-deficient diet. With such heavy withdrawals of enzymes needed to digest an almost-all-cooked diet, it's not hard to see how we become metabolically enzyme-poor even in middle age: heavy withdrawals and skimpy deposits lead to eventual bankruptcy. Unfortunately, the glands and the major organs, including the brain, suffer most from the unnatural digestive drain on the metabolic enzyme potential. Howell shows how the pancreas swells to meet the great demand for its juices while other glands also abnormally adapt, and how the brain actually shrinks on the all-cooked and over-refined diet.

Putting enzymes to work for you is the focus of Chapter 6, in which Dr. Howell explains the enzyme diet, enzyme therapy, and weight reduction techniques using raw calories from enzyme-rich foods. Perhaps this is the first logical attempt to explain the cause of overweight. Howell's solution is equally lucid: the substitution of raw calories for cooked ones as much as possible. Raw milk, bananas, avocados, seeds, nuts, grapes, and many other natural foods are singled out as being moderately high in calories and in food enzymes too. Enzyme supplements are suggsted for use with all cooked foods, and in larger dosages, under supervision, in enzyme therapy.

The question of enzyme inhibitors in raw foods, especially seeds, is put to rest in Chapter 7. For while inhibitors do exist and can block the digestion of food elements by inhibiting enzyme activity, Dr. Howell discusses the best methods of eliminating them from foods altogether.

Finally, Chapters 8 and 9 turn to the problems of allergies and degenerative diseases. Cancer, arthritis, and heart disease are discussed in the light of enzyme therapy, fasting, and raw diets. Here again, the animal kingdom and native cultures provide us with a wealth of information: Whales, which carry a layer of fat up to six inches, yet have completely clean artieries, free of cholesterol; and the Eskimos, who sometimes eat several pounds of fat per day. Yet, medical officers in exploration teams unanimously found clean arteries and no obesity among them. How do the whales and primitive Eskimos escape the ravages of animal fats? Both eat fats raw, with their full complement of lipase, a fat-digesting food enzyme found abundantly in all raw foods containing sizable quantitites of animal or vegetable fat.

The causes of cancer, arthritis, and allergies are equally understandable in light of the Food Enzyme Concept, as are the remedial approaches and preventive measures.

As an author, lecturer, researcher, and former Director of the Hippocrates Health Institute, I have seen remarkable healings and improvements in health and energy levels in individuals following periods on raw food diets. In many cases dramatic results are often obtained within a month or less, especially in problems of toxicity, exhaustion, low energy levels, and overweight. Of course, accounting for the modern pace of life and the weakened human condition, it may be difficult and potentially harmful to adopt a totally raw diet for extended periods. However, Enzyme Nutrition offers a safe and practical alternative: the use of supplemental enzymes in addition to the cooked foods eaten. Under laboratory conditions, certain of these supplemental enzymes are capable of digesting over a million times their weight in cooked food. Does it not make perfect sense to let outside enzymes do some of the work and save your own limited supply of enzymes for the important work of cellular metabolism?

The Food Enzyme Concept of human nutrition is indeed a revelation—one which stands uncontradicted, even in this age of rapid advancement of technology and new methods of testing. Dr. Howell's contribution to the understanding of enzymes and raw food research represents a giant leap forward in the science of nutrition, no less so than the monumental discoveries of vitamins and minerals. It is now up to the many dedicated scientists, health activists, and interested lay persons to apply this new knowledge of enzymes and further the potentials for healing, vibrant health, and longevity that Dr. Howell points to.

Stephen Blauer
Boston, MA

The *length of life* is inversely proportional to the *rate* of exhaustion of the *enzyme potential* of an organism. The increased use of food enzymes promotes a *decreased rate* of exhaustion of the enzyme potential.

The Enzyme Nutrition Axiom
—Dr. Edward Howell

1

Introduction to
Enzyme Nutrition

THE ENZYME COMPLEX

I adhere to the philosophy that both the living organism and its enzymes are inhabited by a vital principle or life energy which is separate and distinct from the caloric energy liberated from food by enzyme action. I would not like to think, when a person talks to me face to face, that it is the energy of the potato he has just digested that is producing his whimsical remarks and animated conversation. I prefer to believe that complex emotions, such as joy, sorrow, and anger, are powered by the same vital energy that the enzyme complex utilizes in metabolizing food—not by the caloric energy of a potato or other food. Emotions are capable of being expressed even in starving persons where there is no food in the body to supply caloric energy.

I define the enzyme complex in biological rather than chemical terms. The enzyme complex harbors a protein carrier inhabited by a vital energy factor. For almost a hundred years chemistry has maintained that enzymes work by their mere presence, without being used up in the process. It has implied that the energy powering enzyme activity is derived, not from the enzymes, but solely from the substrate (the substance being changed or metabolized). If that is true, where does the energy come from to trigger or start the reaction before the energy of the substrate is released to become available? Chemistry concedes that only the living organism can make enzymes, but it implies it can do this without paying a price. Official chemistry maintains, at least by implication, that enzymes are mere chemical flunkies; that they are recklessly expendable. The Food Enzyme Concept holds that organisms endow enzymes with a vital activity factor that is exhaustible. Also that the capacity of a living organism to make enzymes—the enzyme potential—is limited and exhaustible.

The chemical conception that enzymes work by their mere presence, without being used up in the process, is based upon the epochal work of O'Sullivan and Tompson on invertase, published in 1890. Nowhere in this work of almost a hundred pages do the authors state that enzymes work by their mere presence and are not used up in the process. O'Sullivan and Tompson took a tolerant attitude toward the definition of Roberts, Lumlian Lectures (1880), that the living body imparts a definite amount of vital force to enzymes, and that this force acts upon a substrate until it is exhausted.

Enzymes represent the life element which is biologically recognized and can be measured in terms of enzyme activity. Our easiest measurement is a lack, for various chemical reactions fail to occur without enzymes: a radiated or cooked potato will fail to sprout. Thought of for years as catalysts, enzymes are much more than these inert substances. Catalysts work by chemical action only, while enzymes function by both biological and chemical action. Catalysts do not contain the "life element," which is measured as a kind of radiation which enzymes emit. This radiation cannot be measured simply by any ordinary device, but it can be demonstrated by biological means and other methods. The following are means of identifying this hidden entity: The Mitogenetic Rays of Gurwitsch, Kirlian Electro-Magnetic Photography, Rothen's Enzyme Action at a Distance, and Visual Micro Observation of Working Enzymes. Enzymes contain proteins and some contain vitamins which can and have been synthesized by chemists. However, the "life principle" or "activity factor" of the enzyme has never been synthesized. The proteins in enzymes serve merely as carriers of enzyme activity factors. We can summarize that enzymes are protein carriers charged with vital energy factors, just as your car battery consists of metal plates charged with electrical energy. The objectionable idea that enzymes are not exhaustible was coined by others later and ignores the biological evidence that is the topic of this book, *Enzyme Nutrition*.

ENZYMES AND DISEASE

The human race is at least half sick. In a biological sense, there are no completely healthy people living on the conventional diet. Even those young adults who feel fit have health defects. Some have dental caries, thin hair, approaching baldness, acne or allergies, headaches, impaired vision, constipation, and so on, ad infinitum. And these are just superficial phenomena that the individuals can spot themselves. Medical examination finds more. How many ailments afflict the human race? One hundred? Five hundred? One thousand? Are we more expert in breeding disease than are wild animals? Can you name even one species of wild animal afflicted with a hundred diseases? Fifty? Twenty-five? Or even one? We must exclude "wild" animals that feast at our garbage dumps. To make themselves disease-proof, do wild animals perform some special ceremony we don't know about? We shall see.

There are three classes of enzymes: metabolic enzymes, which run our bodies; digestive enzymes, which digest our food; and food enzymes from raw foods, which start food digestion. Our bodies—all our organs and tissues—are run by metabolic enzymes. These enzyme workers take proteins, fats, and carbohydrates (starches, sugars, etc.), and structure them into healthy bodies, keeping everything working properly. Every organ and tissue has its own particular metabolic enzymes to do specialized work. One authority made an investigation and found 98 distinct enzymes working in the arteries, each with a particular job to do. The liver has numerous different enzymes working. No one has ever investigated how many specific enzymes are needed to run the heart, brain, lungs, kidneys, etc.

Since good health depends on all of these metabolic enzymes doing an excellent job, we must be sure that nothing interferes with the body making enough of them. A shortage could mean trouble, many times serious. Modern research is implicating enzymes in all of our activities. Even thinking involves some enzyme activity. In 1930, 80 enzymes were known; in 1947, 200; in 1957, 660; in 1962, 850; and by 1968, science had identified 1300 of them. If you wanted to find out how many enzymes are known today, you might have to hire a specialist full-time to make a survey. And although thousands of enzymes are known, many more reactions have been identified for which the enzymes responsible are not yet known. Hundreds of metabolic enzymes are necessary to carry on the work of the body—to repair damage and decay, and heal diseases.

Digestive enzymes have only three main jobs: digesting protein, carbohydrate, and fat. *Proteases* are enzymes that digest protein; *amylases* digest carbohydrate, and *lipases* digest fat. Nature's plan calls for food enzymes to help with digestion instead of forcing the body's digestive enzymes to carry the whole load. If food enzymes do some of the work, according to the Law of Adaptive Secretion of Digestive

Enzymes, the enzyme potential can allot less activity to digestive enzymes, and have much more to give to the hundreds of metabolic enzymes that run the entire body. If food enzymes did some of the work, the enzyme potential would not be facing impending bankruptcy, as it is now in the bodies of millions of people on the minus diet—food minus its enzymes. Our enzyme potential has a problem somewhat similar to a checking account which could become dangerously deficient if not continually replenished.

THE FOOD ENZYME CONCEPT

The Food Enzyme Concept introduces a new way of looking at disease. It heralds a revolution in our understanding of disease processes. According to the Food Enzyme Concept, enzymes possess biological, as well as chemical, properties. When ingested, the enzymes in raw food, or supplementary enzymes, result in a significant degree of digestion, lowering the drain on the organism's own enzyme potential. The heat used in cooking destroys all food enzymes and forces the organism to produce more enzymes, thus enlarging digestive organs, especially the pancreas. When an excessive amount of digestive enzymes is made, the enzyme potential may be unable to produce an adequate quantity of metabolic enzymes to repair body organs and fight disease. Are digestive enzymes being wasted? The Food Enzyme Concept furnishes conclusive proof that in most people digestive enzymes are being used up with reckless abandon. Although the body makes less than two dozen digestive enzymes, it uses up more of its enzyme potential supplying these than it uses to make the hundreds of metabolic enzymes needed to keep all of the organs and tissues functioning with their diversified activities. The digestive enzymes of civilized humans are infinitely stronger and more concentrated in enzyme activity than any of the metabolic enzymes—more concentrated than any other enzyme combination found in nature. Human saliva and pancreatic juice are loaded with enzyme activity. There is no evidence that wild animals, living on natural raw diets, have digestive enzyme juices even remotely approaching the strength of those found in civilized human beings.

THE LAW OF ADAPTIVE SECRETION
OF DIGESTIVE ENZYMES

If the human organism must devote a huge portion of its enzyme potential to making digestive enzymes, it spells trouble for the whole body because there is a strain on production of metabolic enzymes and there may not be enough enzyme potential to go around. There is competition between the two classes of enzymes. Does science point a way out of this desperate situation? Yes. In 1943, the physiological laboratory of Northwestern University established the Law of Adaptive Secretion of Digestive Enzymes by experiments on rats. The amount of digestive enzymes secreted by the pancreas in response to carbohydrate, protein, and fat was measured and it was found that the strength of each enzyme varied with the amount of each of these food materials it was called upon to digest. Prior to this it was assumed that enzymes were secreted in equal proportions, according to the rule laid down by Professor Babkin. The Law of Adaptive Secretion of Digestive Enzymes holds that the organism values its enzymes highly and will make no more than are needed for the job. If some of the food is digested by enzymes in the food, the body will make less concentrated digestive enzymes. The Law of Adaptive Secretion of Digestive Enzymes has since been confirmed by dozens of university laboratories throughout the world.

If humans take in more exogenous (outside) digestive enzymes, as nature ordained, the enzyme potential will not have to waste so much of its heritage digesting food. It can distribute more of this precious commodity to the metabolic enzymes, where it rightfully belongs. This rightful distribution of enzyme energy will not only act to maintain health and prevent disease, but is expected to help cure established disease. The old saying that nature will cure really refers to metabolic enzyme activity, because there is no other mechanism in the body to cure anything.

To get enzymes from food, one must eat raw food. All life, whether plant or animal, requires the presence of enzymes to keep it going. Therefore, all plant and animal food in the raw state has them. But the mere touch of heat destroys them. Enzymes tolerate no heat at all. They are different from vitamins in this respect. Pasteurization destroys the life force in them, even though much less heat is used than in cooking (145°F versus 300 ° F or higher). If water is hot enough to feel uncomfortable to the hand, it will injure enzymes in food. All foods from a food factory have been heat processed by one means or another.

Evidence of Enzyme Wastage

We are guilty of being careless with enzymes. They are the most precious asset we possess and we should welcome outside enzyme help. If we depend solely upon the enzymes we inherit, they will be used up just like inherited money that is not supplemented by a steady income. The Food Enzyme Concept points out that acute wastage of large quantities of enzymes is strenuously objected to by the body. It can lead to serious illness and even death. In an experiment in 1944, young rats and chickens were fed a diet of raw soybeans (high in enzyme inhibitors) and huge quantities of pancreatic digestive enzymes were wasted in combating the inhibitors. The pancreas gland enlarged to handle the extra burden, and the animals sickened and failed to grow. Soybeans are seeds, and all seeds have some enzyme inhibitors. (Enzyme inhibitors are discussed in Chapter 7.) The early experiments, proving that organisms rebel against having their enzymes wasted, have now been repeated and amplified in dozens of scientific experimental laboratories. Eating the seeds and their inhibitors causes a great outpouring and wastage of pancreatic digestive enzymes, enlargement of the pancreas, decrease in the supply of metabolic enzymes, stunted growth, and impaired health.

My organ weight tables, some of which are presented in this book (see pp. 81, 126), show that the size and weight of the pancreas varies with the type of diet. When the pancreas must process more enzymes, it enlarges. Is this wholesome for the individual? When the heart works too hard pumping blood through damaged arteries, it enlarges. Who wants an enlarged heart? Are enlarged tonsils something to desire? Or an enlarged thyroid gland, turning into a goiter? What about an enlarged liver? The everyday variety of enlarged pancreas is painless, not letting its owner know it is doing anything wrong, while indiscriminately handling the enzyme activity doled out to it and stressing the whole system. We are guilty of forcing our precious enzyme activity to do all of the menial work of digestion and then expect it also to do a perfect job on the metabolism. Food enzymes, and other exogenous enzymes, can help with digestion, but not with metabolism. Then why not let these helper-enzymes free our body's energy stores to more efficiently run the metabolism of the body?

Animals such as cattle and sheep get along with a pancreas about a third as large as ours (figured as a percentage of the body weight) on their raw food diet. Laboratory mice, eating the standard laboratory chow diet of heat-processed, enzyme-free food, have a pancreas two to three times heavier than that of wild mice eating the enzyme diet of raw food they find in nature. When laboratory rats are put on an enzyme-rich diet of raw food, their pancreas gets only about one third as heavy as the same gland in rats fed a random diet, or one totally free of enzymes.

The tremendous impact that wastage of body enzymes can have on health and even life itself is pointed out by experiments performed on animals. At Washington University, surgeons equipped a group of dogs with fistulae (tubes) designed to drain all of the pancreatic juice enzymes out of the body and waste them. Despite the animals' usual access to food and water, profound deterioration set in, and all of them died within a week. This experiment was later duplicated on rats by other research workers and the same sequence of events took place, with death following in less than a week. Acute human intestinal obstruction has been described as resulting in death within three to five days. Both in experimental intestinal obstruction in the dog, and in spontaneous human obstruction, authorities believe death is attributable to loss of pancreatic juice enzymes, caused by continuous vomiting. It is a remarkable fact that prolonged loss of bile through biliary fistulae, which prevent bile from entering the intestines, is not fatal in man or in laboratory animals, because no enzymes are wasted in this instance. The modern human digestive system makes extravagant demands on the enzyme potential. In this area man is in a class by himself, unlike all of nature's creatures in the wild. Indeed, only humans live on enzyme-free food. All wild creatures get their enzyme supplements in the raw food itself. Animals using raw food do not have the rich concentrations of enzyme activity in their digestive juices that humans do. Many animals have no enzymes at all in the saliva. But human saliva is loaded with a fantastically high concentration of the enzyme amylase, also known as ptyalin. Cattle and sheep secrete huge quantities of saliva entirely devoid of enzymes. The horse has no salivary enzymes on its natural raw diet. When dogs and cats eat their natural raw, carnivorous diet, there are no enzymes in the saliva. But when dogs are fed on a high carbohydrate, heat-treated diet, enzymes show up in the saliva within about a week, obeying the Law of Adaptive Secretion of Digestive Enzymes.

THE FOOD-ENZYME STOMACH

One would think that because ruminants such as cattle and sheep have no enzymes in the saliva, they would have an extra large concentration of enzymes in the pancreatic juice to make up for it. But this is not the case. My organ weight research has, in fact, disclosed that the pancreas of cattle and sheep is much smaller than ours, figured as a percentage of body weight. This shows that these animals get along with far less pancreatic enzymes than we. Cattle and sheep have four stomachs, only one of which secretes enzymes. And this one is the smallest. The other three, which are forestomachs, and which I have named food-enzyme stomachs, have no enzymes of their own, but allow enzymes of the food to digest it. In addition, the forestomachs of ruminants harbor protozoa, giving these tiny animals "free room and board" in exchange for use of the enzymes in digesting the food. It is a nice symbiotic relationship. As the digestion of a meal is advanced, most of the protozoa pass on into the fourth stomach where they are digested and supply a considerable portion of the protein requirements of the ruminants. This raises the question whether animals, such as cattle and sheep, are true vegetarians, since protozoa are animals, and their hosts depend on them for some of their nutrients.

Besides the forestomachs of ruminants, a study of comparative anatomy furnishes other examples of what I have called the food-enzyme stomach. For years, physiologists were puzzled as to the function of these organs. The largest food-enzyme stomach in the world is owned by the whale, the first of three stomachs of this largest member of the Cetacea. The smaller cetaceans are dolphins and porpoises, which also have a food-enzyme stomach and two other stomachs. These food-enzyme stomachs are loaded up with enormous catches of aquatic prey. One killer whale was found to have 32 seals piled up in its food-enzyme stomach. It must be kept in mind that these food-enzyme stomachs secrete no enzymes or acid. How do you suppose this huge pile of whole animals can be broken down to a consistency small enough to pass through the small opening connecting the food-enzyme stomach to the second stomach without enzymes to do the job? Physiologists have also asked this question and several papers from physiologists in different countries have recently appeared in scientific literature trying to resolve this riddle.

The Food Enzyme Concept is the only answer. Each of the 32 seals inside the whale has its own digestive enzymes in its stomach and pancreatic juices. When the whale swallows the seal, these digestive enzymes become the property of the whale. They are now its food enzymes and work for the benefit of the whale during the many days required to digest and empty the contents of the food-enzyme stomach. In addition, all animals have a proteolytic enzyme known as cathepsin, which is widely distributed in muscles and organs, yet has no known digestive function in life. After death, the body tissues become acidic, which is favorable for catheptic activity. This enzyme then functions as the prime factor in autolysis, the breakdown of cells and tissues.

Another example of the food-enzyme stomach is the crop of birds using seeds as food, such as the chicken and pigeon. Physiologists had always stated that the crop has no known function, but that was before the Food Enzyme Concept brought together a consortium of facts to permit a new and more mature outlook. The crop has no enzymes of its own, but all seeds have a good inventory of them. It has been demonstrated that during the sojourn of 10 to 15 hours that intact seeds remain in the crop, they accumulate moisture; their enzymes multiply; there is incipient germination; enzyme inhibitors are neutralized, and starch is digested to dextrin and maltose. This digestion in the food-enzyme stomach (crop) by food enzymes is continued when the crop contents are emptied into the gizzard, and perhaps further along in the gastrointestinal tract. It becomes evident that in many animals, perhaps all, provision has been made for the digestion of food by food enzymes. Is the human being included?

FOOD ENZYME DIGESTION IN HUMANS

According to the Food Enzyme Concept, there is a mechanism operating in all creatures permitting food enzymes to digest a particular fraction of the food in whch they are contained. In humans, the upper portion of the stomach is in fact a food-enzyme stomach. This part secretes no enzymes. It behaves the same as other food-enzyme stomachs. When raw food with its enzymes is eaten, it goes into this peristalsis-free food-enzyme section of our stomach where these food enzymes digest the food. In fact, the digestion of the protein, carbohydrate, and fat in raw food begins in the mouth at the very moment the plant cell walls are ruptured, releasing the food enzymes during the act of mastication. After swallowing, digestion continues in the food-enzyme section of the stomach for one-half to one hour, or until the rising tide of acidity reaches a point where it is inhibited. Then the stomach enzyme pepsin takes over.

Once food is swallowed, it settles in a mass in the food-enzyme section of our stomachs. If it is cooked, enzyme-free food, it waits there for a period of one-half to one hour, during which time nothing happens to it. If harmful bacteria are swallowed with the food they may attack it during this time of enforced idleness. The salivary enzyme works on the carbohydrate, but the protein and fat must wait.

Here is where proper enzyme digestive supplements fit in. Taken and chewed up with the meal, these exogenous digestive enzymes begin immediate digestion of all nutrients. They work on the protein, carbohydrate, and fat during the half-hour to hour period that these foods remain in the food-enzyme part of the stomach. According to the Law of Adaptive Secretion of Digestive Enzymes, whatever digestion is accomplished by enzyme supplements or food enzymes does not have to be done by the digestive enzymes of the body. There is no further need for such rich digestive enzyme juices. This desirable reaction results in a conservation of the enzyme potential and body energy. It allows the body to devote its attention to supplying more metabolic enzymes for use by the organs and tissues to carry on their functions, provide repairs, and bring about cures.

RESEARCH FINDINGS

Let us check the Law of Adaptive Secretion of Digestive Enzymes against research findings. Some people believe that the low pH of the human stomach stops most of the digestive activity of salivary, and, presumably, supplemental enzymes, because the pH (measurement of the acidity or alkalinity of a solution) of human saliva is neutral (7). It can be seen, however, that salivary amylase does assist in digestion in the stomach, and that food and supplemental enzymes are even more effective.

Olaf Bergeim, professor of physiology at Illinois College of Medicine, reported his research on gastric salivary digestion of starch with 12 dental students as subjects. Bergeim stressed that starch digestion cannot be studied *in vitro* (in the laboratory), but that the investigation must be done on specimens of material that have been removed from the living stomach after undergoing digestion. His results showed that an average of 76 percent of the starch of mashed potatoes, and 59 percent of the starch of bread was converted to maltose, and an additional percentage was changed to dextrose. Bergeim quoted Muller, who used rice cereal as a test meal on human subjects and found 59 to 80 percent of the carbohydrate was rendered soluble, and 50 to 77 percent of the starch in bread was made soluble when human subjects ate test meals. Professor Bergeim aspirated the digested food from the stomach after 45 minutes, but concluded that even 15 minutes in the stomach allowed time for significant digestion. The subjects were instructed to masticate the food thoroughly, which ensured initial digestion by saliva even before the food was swallowed. The professor explained experiments he made *in vitro* in which hydrochloric acid, a chemical present in stomach juices, was added to saliva and caused permanent inactivation. However, investigations by others have since shown that the average human secretions of hydrochloric acid are not as concentrated as was believed. This not only allows more stomach digestion to occur by salivary amylase and exogenous enzymes, but permits more reactivation of the enzymes after the stomach contents become neutralized in the alkaline duodenum. More recent experiments conducted in Europe *in vivo* (in the living organism) found that salivary amylase and supplemental enzymes were recovered in the duodenum and lower in the intestine, showing that supplemental enzymes and food enzymes may be reactivated by the juices of the intestine.

Research by Dr. Beazell reported in the *Journal of Laboratory and Clinical Medicine*, 1941, and the *American Journal of Physiology*, 1941, holds more information. Using 11 normal, young adult males, Beazell found that the human stomach digested several times more starch than protein at the end of an hour. Therefore he felt that the emphasis placed on the stomach as an organ for protein digestion is misplaced, because the stomach digests more starch than protein. Furthermore, if the salivary amylase can digest considerable starch at a pH no lower than 5 or 6, how much protein, fat, and starch can food enzymes or supplemental enzymes digest, since their range for activity extends down even below 3 in some instances?

The foregoing evidence clearly establishes that a large quantity of starch is regularly digested in the human stomach by salivary amylase, even though it is not the ideal enzyme to work in the stomach. Where, then, do critics get the authority to state that food enzymes and supplemental enzymes do not digest food in the stomach? Reading such statements in textbooks is misleading. They may merely be the opinions of the authors, unless they are shown to be based on actual research work that is recorded in scientific periodical literature. What is to prevent food enzymes and supplemental enzymes, with better pH credentials than salivary amylase, from digesting even more protein, fat, and carbohydrate in the stomach?

Work done at the laboratory of physiology at Northwestern University bears heavily on the quantity of supplemental enzymes passing through the stomach uninjured. In the *Journal of Nutrition*, A. C. Ivy, C. R. Schmitt, and J. M. Beazell showed by experiments on humans that an average of 51 percent of malt amylase, an enzyme produced by germinating barley, passed into the intestine in active form, after it had digested starch in the stomach. In human subjects, malt amylase augmented the digestion of starch when a deficiency of salivary secretion was simulated. It must be remembered that the subjects used were healthy, young males and not older adults deficient in salivary amylase. The Food Enzyme Concept holds that human digestive fluids have an unacceptably high enzyme content, much richer than those of wild creatures. There are indications that this anomaly may impede production of hundreds of specific metabolic enzymes needed for diverse metabolic chores. The digestive secretions of humans in the prime of life are pathologically rich, at the expense of metabolic enzymes. In a set of experiments on human subjects, it was found that the average strength of salivary amylase was 30 times higher in a group of younger adults than in a group of older adults.

Dr. W. H. Taylor, University of Oxford, investigated the optimal pH at which the stomach digested protein *in vitro*. Surprisingly, he found not one, but *two* zones of maximal activity. One was pH 1.6 to 2.4, at which the enzyme pepsin is active. The other zone extended from pH 3.3 to 4.0, where cathepsin acts. It was found that the amount of protein digestion taking place at each zone was approximately equal. This meant that pepsin is not the only enzyme performing stomach digestion, but that cathepsin does an equal amount of work in digesting meat and vegetable proteins.

Animal flesh and organs, particularly muscle meat, are amply provided with cathepsin. It is found in every pound of meat in the butcher shop. When a tiger or other carnivore tears off chunks of flesh from his prey and swallows them, the cathepsin within the meat itself is right at home, and lightens the burden of digestion for its counterpart in the warm confines of the stomach, because it operates at precisely the same pH. If it is conceded that there are no reasons why the food enzyme cathepsin should not engage in gastric digestion equally with the cathepsin secreted by the stomach, on what grounds should other food enzymes with like pH characteristics be disqualified from participating in gastric digestion? Gastric cathepsin and food cathepsin operate at pH 3 to 4. Amylases in wheat and other grains also function well at pH 3 to 4. Various vegetable proteases and lipases likewise operate in this range. How can these food enzymes be prevented from digesting food substrates in the human stomach, when nature has provided the ideal gastric pH environment for them to digest protein, carbohydrate, and fat?

ENZYME NUTRITION

Raw food does not stimulate enzyme secretion as much as cooked food. Less stomach acid is secreted. This permits food enzymes to operate for a longer period in the food-enzyme section of the stomach than when the meal consists of cooked food. Consequently, more digestion is performed by food enzymes. When food enzymes, or other exogenous enzymes are permitted to do more work, this results in normalizing and lessening the strength of excessively high digestive enzyme secretions, such as pancreatic juice and saliva. Food enzymes are much less concentrated than pancreatic digestive enzymes. Digestion of a raw food meal takes more time. When a jungle lion finishes a meal, its stomach is full of large chunks of raw meat, perhaps 30 or more pounds. A period of stupor sets in, during which time cathepsin within the meat starts digesting it. Later, pepsin from the lion's stomach juice digests the meat chunks from the outside, while the food enzymes continue to digest them from within. Several days may pass before the job is completed. When a small snake swallows a frog, or when a large snake like a python swallows a pig, a big distention appears in the body of the snake in the area of the stomach, and the same events transpire. The cathepsin of the prey and its digestive enzymes now become the food enzymes of the snake host and work for its benefit. There is nothing to prevent the digestive enzymes of the prey from doing the same job in the stomach of their new owner as they did during life for the benefit of their former owner. It may require a week for the food enzymes, plus the snake's digestive enzymes, to digest the meal and make the distention disappear.

Careful study shows that nature's creatures possess a food-enzyme stomach or its equivalent that allows their exclusively raw food diet to be predigested, relieving their digestive organs of excess work. Humans also possess a food-enzyme stomach which, as we have shown, is capable of relieving the digestive burden when food enzymes are included in the diet. In the chapters that follow, I will explain the role of food enzymes in health and show how we can harness their energy-giving properties for healing, greater health, and longer life. I will also cover their application in the treatment of various degenerative illnesses affecting mankind today.

2

Food Enzymes Add Life

CAUSES OF DISEASE

Enzyme Nutrition and the Food Enzyme Concept may have more to offer as a permanent contribution to those seeking health than any system yet proposed. The Food Enzyme Concept points out the basic, underlying causes of the killer diseases and seeks to eradicate these causes, as a supplement to palliative emergency measures.

Many of the intractable diseases have two causes. The first is the chief culprit: enzyme deficiency or undernutrition, the all-important, underlying, hidden predisposing first cause. It works in your body by setting the stage, preparing the ground, and acting behind the scenes, painlessly, silently, and treacherously. The Food Enzyme Concept reveals how the mechanism of enzyme deficiency speeds the development of cancer, heart disease, arthritis, premature aging and other intractable conditions.

The second more highly advertised "cause" of disease can bring out trouble only if the first has done its work well. It comprises such mischief-makers as carcinogens, cholesterol, bacteria, X-rays, food additives, and tobacco smoke. Smoking only acts to stimulate disease, as a spark which can grow into a flame and burn out an already unhealthy body. We all know people who have smoked for a lifetime without developing cancer. Similarly, millions of persons have used saccharin and food additives, have been exposed to X-rays, have drunk polluted water and breathed polluted air, and yet appear to be immune to the toxic properties of these agents. This is not to say that I condone polluting the body with harmful materials. But I contend that those individuals getting more enzyme reinforcements from outside sources have better tools to deal with these damaging substances than those who have no such reinforcements.

COOKING DESTROYS ENZYMES

How does the Food Enzyme Concept explain the cause of killer and intractable diseases—ailments that refuse to go away? These are the maladies that medical textbooks have always branded with the stigma "etiology unknown." I attest that the kitchen stove and its big brothers, the heat-treatment machinery in food factories, are responsible for destroying a whole category of food elements, namely the heat-sensitive, exogenous food enzymes. These nutritional supplements have always provided our endogenous (internal) enzymes with the enzyme reinforcements needed to check the disease-making process.

High temperatures, as in cooking, destroy enzymes in natural foods. But, I can almost hear you say, "This cannot be, because the human race has been cooking for a long time and is still going strong." Partly true. We are only half sick. What poses as good health today has been aptly termed by one doctor as "pregnant ill-health," or the absence of symptoms. Good health as we know it is in reality a prolonged incubation period for a variety of killer and intractable diseases. No matter from which angle we view health and disease, we cannot escape from being entangled in the conclusion that intractable disease is as old as cookery. Disease and cookery originated simultaneously. And cookery must be held guilty of assassinating hundreds of food enzymes which, we must be constantly reminded, are the most delicate and precious elements that foods can offer us.

If you still have some doubt that the present essentially enzymeless diet is the parent or grandparent of a multitude of our health problems, let me present some evidence. That we cannot be elated over the status of the nation's health is shown by the enormous cost of medical and hospital care, and by the huge variety of drugs displayed in stores and advertised in the media. Contrast this consequence of undernutrition with the condition of any group of wild animals you wish to name; living in the deep jungle, under the ocean or in the air. Animals subsist on raw, natural food with enzymes—not cooked food.

Wild Animals Are Healthy

Have you ever heard of a racing ambulance speeding through the jungle with siren screaming, rushing a valuable wild lion to a hospital with a heart attack? Has any hunter or animal observer ever seen a wild elephant, or any jungle inhabitant, hobbling along painfully on deformed arthritic joints? A wild female chimpanzee or gorilla with a breast eaten into by cancer would make newspaper headlines all over the world. We expect these denizens of the wild to be free of all disease. Let us not lose sight of the fact that the reason they are disease-free is due to their superb enzyme nutrition. Among the many thousands of species of creatures living on this earth, only humans and some of their domestic animals try to live without food enzymes. And only these transgressors of nature's laws are penalized with defective health. We cannot ascribe poor human health to vitamin or mineral deficiencies because foods have been fortified to the hilt with these.

It has been suggested that wild animals are free from the stress of civilized life, and this is the reason they escape our ailments. They do not have to worry about paying rent or taxes. They are not exposed to the stress of working long hours and do not have our worries and frustrations. This philosophy of stress as an etiological (causative) factor in human disease has been blown out of all proportion to reality. If you feel it is hard to cope with life under civilization, how would you like to trade places with grazing animals in the wild, whose only defense against fierce predators is speedy flight? Stress from various sources—ecological, increasing human population, etc., is slowly overtaking animals, too. Here is another example.

Consider the wild city rat, with dogs, cats, and angry humans bent on killing it on sight, or a wild rodent in the field that cannot leave its burrow without facing attack from lurking predators on the ground or sharp-eyed hawks in the air. The potential prey must experience the height of tension trying to prolong its life, while plagued by constant fear that it may end at any moment. On the other hand, the predators also must bring into play a great degree of tension to get a meal or face starvation. It can be seen that among wild creatures the ability to muster a high level of tension is now a matter involving life and death. Humans are exposed to less physical tension, yet we not only have inferior health, but display disfiguring degenerative diseases as well. Thus the stress theory appears to leak at the seams and cannot hold water.

There is little doubt that modern emotional stress can potentially affect health and the stress theory might be accepted as representing a minor, contributing, secondary cause of human disease, a so-called exciting cause. However, the basic, primary cause remains nutritional deficiency, and enzyme undernutrition must be rated high. Advocates might try to rescue the stress theory by suggesitng that humans have to contend more with chronic stress, instead of the acute variety. The stress reaction in man and animal results when stimuli cause the adrenal glands to secrete the hormone adrenalin, which in turn stimulates the heart, increases blood pressure, and brings sugar into the blood. These reactions are necessary to enable an animal under attack by a predator to start a rapid getaway in an attempt to save its life. They also trigger a predator to even greater action to win a meal and prevent possible starvation.

But when the stress reaction becomes habitual in human beings in response to many diverse, annoying or exasperating situations arising in the course of a day, a chronic state of hypertension may arise. This may involve the heart and nervous system, and arterial hypertension, eventually spilling over and producing various and diverse symptoms. Or so the theory goes.

However, when we try to accept the stress-reaction syndrome as a cause of disease, a contradiction crops up. If we place heavy emphasis upon stress as a primary cause of various diseases, and ignore the role played by undernutrition, it could be expected that wild animals would display a larger incidence of disease than humans, because the stress reaction in wild animals must be so taxing and consuming as to spell the difference between life and death. But we all know the reverse is true. Wild creatures of the deep jungle are essentially free of disease. A basic difference between wild and laboratory rats is shown by the iron nerves of wild rats fighting an experimentally produced irritating sound, in contrast to laboratory rats that give up and die.

The contradiction becomes still wider when it is realized that wild animals secrete much more adrenalin than their domesticated cousins. This information is supplied by comparing the weight of the adrenal glands of wild animals with those of captive animals such as laboratory specimens used in research. Captive tame animals are protected from predators and therefore have no need to resort to the stress reaction triggered by adrenalin, and so adrenalin output drops and the adrenal glands become smaller. This is dramatically illustrated in Table 2.1. It shows that in wild rats the adrenal glands are almost twice as large as in the tame variety, while in wild mice the adrenals are more than twice as large as in their tame cousins.

Table 2.1

COMPARISON OF WEIGHT OF ADRENAL GLANDS
WILD AND LABORATORY FEMALE RODENTS

Subjects	Adrenals as % of Body Weight
Laboratory Rats	0.0257
Wild Rats	0.0471
Laboratory Mice	0.0295
Wild Mice	0.0675

Abridged from my organ weight tables. Expressed as percent of 100 grams of body weight.

This data could suggest that because wild rats and wild mice have larger adrenal glands, which produce more adrenalin, the wild creatures should have more disease than the tame ones. But since the very reverse is true, it is obvious that the stress theory is in trouble. By weighing the factors involved, there is no alternative to the conclusion that the stress theory cannot account for the primary cause of disease. That the primary cause of most disease is undernutrition has been amply demonstrated by research, and enzyme undernutrition stands out as a prime architect of this health bankruptcy.

ENZYMES CAN AND DO WEAR OUT

Now let us deal with the allegations in encyclopedias, dictionaries, and textbooks that enzymes work by their mere presence and are not used up in doing their jobs. This is an outrageous declaration and leads to the dangerous expectation that, by some special kind of magic, the enzyme checking account cannot be overdrawn and will last forever. This false but "official" doctrine deceives even the best-intentioned doctors and other technical people. If a doctor believes this myth which leads to falsifying the behavior of enzymes, he will not recognize the early warning signs of enzyme undernutrition and bankruptcy. I feel it is necessary to submit more related evidence to offset the "official" concept of enzymes.

There are many reports on enzymes in the scientific periodical literature of the world that have not been incorporated into the textbooks by professors and instructors to teach their students in our colleges and universities. I have collected some of this research in my previous work *Food Enzymes for Health and Longevity* first published by the National Enzyme Company in 1946 under the title *The Status of Food Enzymes in Digestion and Metabolism*. That is over thirty-five years ago. This reveals how much time is needed to digest research and put the result into textbooks where students can read it. Why is the term "food enzyme" not even mentioned in textbooks and encyclopedias? The research I have collected presents an avalanche of evidence against the pronouncements in reference books. In contrast, enzymes are used up by all of the varied activities of the organism.

The famous researcher and statistician, Professor Pearl, of Johns Hopkins University, summarized his laborious and important experiments on the duration of life in these words: "In general, duration of life varies inversely with the rate of energy expenditure during its continuance. In short, the length of life depends inversely on the rate of living."

The scientific team MacArthur and Baille of the University of Toronto, at the conclusion of a piece of research, stated:

The organism appears to receive a specific sum total of "vitality" rather than a definite allotment of days. Life runs out its course to its natural term with a velocity directly proportional to the catabolic rate, or, as commonly expressed, according to rapidity of "wear and tear."

Catabolic rate translates into enzyme activity, and wear and tear into enzyme loss. Boiled down, these definitions of life mean that each child is born with a definite amount of enzyme potential. It can be either saved or wasted; used up rapidly by living at a fast tempo, or used sparingly at a slower pace. The enzyme potential can be made to last longer when outside enzyme reinforcements (supplements or raw foods) are taken in.

I wish to quote from my earlier publication, *The Status of Food Enzymes in Digestion and Metabolism*:

It is no longer warranted to consider vitality and life energy as intangible forces. The available evidence does not justify a placid continuance of a nihilistic attitude toward the vital forces operating in the living organism. Enzymes emerge as the true yardstick of vitality. Enzymes offer an important means of calculating the vital energy of an organism. That which has ben referred to as vitality, vital force, vital energy, vital activity, nerve energy, nerve force, strength, vital resistance, life energy, life and life force, may be, and probably is, synonymous with that which has been known as enzyme activity, enzyme value, enzyme energy, enzyme vitality and enzyme content.

In the year 1958, I devised a method of capturing enzyme activity on film by motion picture microphotography. The description and plates shown in Figure 2.1 are reproduced by permission of the National Enzyme Company. The action shows how the plant enzyme amylase dismantles the starch cell (granule) in less than a minute through a series of remarkable transformatons. If you still have only a vague idea of what enzyme action is, you should see the film *Motion Picture Microphotography of Enzyme Action*, which is available through the National Enzyme Company.

Table 2.1

MOTION PICTURE MICROPHOTOGRAPHY OF ENZYME ACTION

Experiment Number 2

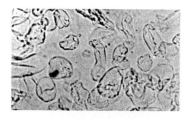
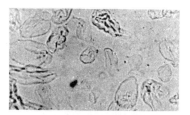

Plant amylase added.   After 12 seconds digestion.

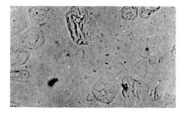
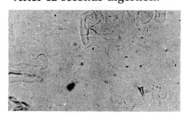

After 23 seconds digestion.   After 35 seconds digestion.

The strength of enzymes can be analyzed and has been routinely analyzed and measured in the laboratory. The evidence I shall present, plus evidence tabulated in my former volume, makes it abundantly clear that the so-called "life force" or vitality can be measured by laboratory methods, since these entities can be equated with enzyme activity. This evidence also establishes that the enzyme complex not only carries protein, but that this protein is impregnated and inhabited by a vital component that may be called the enzyme potential. Furthermore, the evidence suggests that enzyme supplements should be used just as faithfully as vitamin and mineral supplements, particularly when people cannot or will not take these nutrients as nature offers them in food.

Unless I wish to shut my mind and live in an unreal world, I must conclude that the books used in libraries and schools of higher learning are incomplete, because they present only a chemical and not a biological conception of enzymes.

But the statement that enzymes act by their mere presence and are never used up by the work they do has been repeated for more than 75 years the world over in thousands of books. It so thoroughly stains the fabric of scientific thought that it may require a couple of lifetimes to clean it out.

Enzymes at Varied Temperatures

We have already seen that the high temperatures commonly used in cooking destroy enzymes. But another remarkable fact about enzymes is that they do more work at *slightly* warmer temperatures than they do at cooler ones. For instance, an experiment digesting starch outside of the body may be performed by placing equal amounts of soluble potato starch into each of two dishes, and adding the same amount of water and saliva to each. Saliva contains the enzyme amylase, also known as ptyalin. One dish may be placed in a warm room at about 80° F, and the other dish in the refrigerator at about 40° F. With the proper equipment it can be demonstrated that the starch at room temperature would be digested rapidly, whereas digestion would be feeble at the refrigerator temperature.

If one wanted to go further and put a dish of the starch-enzyme mixture in a room with a temperature of 100° F, the enzymes would do at least four times as much work as at 80°. At 120 ° they could accomplish eight times as much as at 80 °. At 160°, they could do more than 16 times as much. But at 160° F, the enzymes wear out in about a half-hour and can no longer do any work. Some industries take advantage of the capacity of enzymes to work harder as the temperature goes up—it speeds up production in factories. They have automatic conveying systems that carry their products through various enzyme baths at high temperatures, replacing the worn-out enzymes at short intervals. They can afford the added cost of the enzyme replacement in the interest of higher production. What I wish to emphasize in this connection is that while enzymes do more work with increasing temperatures, they are used up faster. This refutes the pronouncement of encyclopedias and textbooks that enzymes are not used up.

Official chemistry will tell you that 160° F denatures (changes the nature of) the protein in enzymes. But that does not explain why enzymes do more work in a dish, test tube or continuous industrial bath at high temperatures. Chemistry cannot explain this, but biology can. When the temperature of a living organism is raised, the enzymes within work faster than at the normal temperature. This has a special value in a feverish condition associated with a bacterial infection. The increased temperature in a fever induces faster enzyme action, and hence is unfavorable for bacterial action. The numerous varieties of hungry enzymes frequenting white blood cells are overwhelming during a fever and often, if the fever is left alone, the white blood cells will make short work of the germs by engulfing and digesting them through the mechanism called phagocytosis.

Therefore, we must conclude that a fever is often necessary, and taking aspirin or other drugs to suppress it may be the worst thing to do. If the fever is high, you had better let the professional doctor make the decision. The extra work enzymes do during a fever causes some of them to wear out to an extent that the system expels them through the urine. Many tests have found various enzymes in the urine, not only after fevers, but after any athletic activity of a strenuous nature. This wear and tear (all machines, including the living organism, undergo wear and tear) is an attribute of function or living. Here again we have evidence that enzymes wear out and are discarded without denaturation of their protein.

The waste products and "spent" fractions of proteins, carbohydrates, fats, vitamins, minerals, and enzymes are excreted as feces, urine, and sweat, as well as by the lungs, after serving as food. Enzymes do indeed become used up and worn out. They are excreted through the urine and sweat along with other "spent" substances. Many thousands of urine tests have found these used-up enzymes in urine. They are below par and not good enough to retain in the body. All other food elements are replaced daily through food reinforcements. There is a mistaken notion in some quarters that reinforcements of food enzymes, or enzyme supplements, are not needed because the body can make its own enzymes. Laboratory research confirms that it is self-defeating to obligate the body to produce excessive amounts of highly concentrated digestive enzymes, due to the drain this places on the rest of the system.

Enzyme Activity and Length of Life

We have learned from a simple experiment how heat makes enzymes work harder and wear out sooner. Now let us see how heat and cold affect enzymes in the living body, which in turn affects its lifespan. The best way to demonstrate this is through the use of small animals called *Daphnia* (the water flea), living in ponds, swamps, and shallow lakes, and serving as food for small fish. These creatures are visible to the naked eye and have a transparent covering that permits viewing the beating of the heart and the movement of the intestines. Being cold-blooded, their lifespan varies with the temperature of the surroundings, which is one reason they are chosen for lifespan research. In warm-blooded animals the temperature of the blood remains fairly constant in hot or cold weather, whereas in cold-blooded creatures the blood approaches the temperature of the environment, within certain limits.

In the experiment, one animal is placed in a small jar containing water and food. A series of such jars is deposited in a bath controlled to maintain a chosen temperature. The animals are monitored until all are dead. The average length of life is then calculated for this particular temperature. A separate experiment must be performed for each temperature. Such experiments were performed by the research team of MacArthur and Baille, University of Toronto, on *Daphnia magna*. These tests are of great value—I can testify because I have done similar work with *Daphnia magna*. The results obtained by MacArthur and Baille appear in Table 2.2.

Table 2.2

LIFESPAN GOVERNED BY SPEED OF ENZYME USE

Temperature		Duration of Life
Degrees F	*Degrees C*	*Days*
46	8	108.2
50	10	87.8
64	18	40.0
82	28	25.6

At the coolest temperature, 46° F, the *Daphnia* lived 108 days, their movements were sluggish, and their heart rate was less than 2 beats per second. At the warmest temperature, 82° F, the animals lived only about 26 days, but their movements were very brisk and their heart rate was almost 7 beats per second.

Frisky Enzymes Are Used Up Sooner

It is plain that at the warm temperature, the metabolic enzymes had a great deal of work to do to keep the animals swimming at a frisky pace, to keep the heart beating very fast, and to perform other body functions associated with living at a speedy tempo. Consequently, their enzymes were worn out in 26 days, at which point life ended. At the cool temperature, the metabolic enzymes had much less work because the animals were languid, their heart rates only about one-third as high, and their associated body functions were done at a correspondingly slower pace than at the warm temperature. As a result their enzyme potential did not wear thin until day 108, which marked the termination of their lifespan. Quoting MacArthur and Baille: "Duration of life varies inversely with the intensity of the metabolism."

What do we learn from this experiment? Simply this: no matter what kind of effort you put forth, be it little or much, you are using up enzymes. A lot of very hard work means more enzymes will go down the drain. To prevent this enzyme loss from shortening the lifespan, we have only one solution—we must provide enzyme reinforcements from the outside to cut down the secretion of digestive enzymes and allow the body to make enough metabolic enzymes.

Make Regular Deposits to Your Enzyme Bank Account

The *Daphnia* research confirms again that enzymes do not just hang around, and by their mere presence, issue a magical command which causes work to be done without laying a hand on it. This credo is professed by sources the public looks to for accurate information. But the experimental work shows the enzymes actually *perform* the work, and *are used up*, and *become worn out* in the process. Furthermore it is shown that when the enzyme potential is exhausted beyond a particular point, it triggers the end of the lifespan. The researchers calaculated that about 15,000,000 heart beats occur during the course of the *Daph-*

nia's lifespan, regardless of whether it lives 26 days with a heart rate of 7 beats per second, or 108 days at 2 beats per second. The organism has a fixed total of enzyme activity to expend. All of these events proceed in strict obeyance to Rubner's Law,* which makes it inexcusable for any further procrastination in accepting the Food Enzyme Concept as a basis for explaining intractable disease and its proper management. Most people spend their enzyme bank account and seldom make a deposit. It would be wiser to conserve enzymes and get enzyme reinforcements from the outside, since various experiments have taught us that enzymes are precious commodities.

Life Ends When Enzymes Get Tired

Official chemistry likes to maintain that the harmful effect heat has on enzymes is due to denaturation of their protein, and shies away from the biological responses to temperature changes. It cannot explain why enzymes work harder in a test tube at 80° F than at 40° F (and also wear out sooner). Or why cold-blooded animals are frisky at 80° F and sluggish at 40° F, and die sooner at 80° F. In both instances the same enzyme mechanism operates and it imparts new meaning to the contention that life is an enzyme process, ending when the enzyme potential becomes depleted beyond a certain point. Can chemistry explain this in terms of protein denaturization?

Strength of Enzyme Potential Fixes Lifespan

I fully realize it may be difficult for many readers to digest and evaluate the various elements of the Food Enzyme Concept and whether or not it leads to a logical conclusion. As I have been agitating for the Food Enzyme Concept for many years, I have no alternative but to offer proof in the form of many separate fractions to establish a whole. At this point I must bring out another facet bearing on the intimate relationship of the enzyme potential to the lifespan. The rating of the enzyme potential determines not only the length of life, but how effectively the organism can maintain a high state of health and deal with disease.

---

*Max Rubner, a German chemist, wrote "Das Problem der Lebens Dauer" ("The Problem of Life's Duration"), which states that the duration of an organism's life has an inverse relationship to its expenditure of energy.

Human Enzymes Weak and Worn Out in Old Age

How strong are the enzymes in the body at the prime of life compared to old age? They should be weak in old age. Put in terms acceptable to the scientific community, it could be said that enzyme activity becomes weaker in old age. Dr. Meyer and his associates at Michael Reese Hospital, Chicago, found that the enzyme of the saliva in young adults was 30 times stronger than in persons over 69 years old. Dr. Eckardt in Germany tested 1,200 urine specimens for the starch-digesting enzyme amylase. In young people it averaged 25 of his test units, and in old people, 14. There are a large number of reports in my files from the scientific periodical literature describing how to increase the lifespan in *Daphnia*, fruit flies, rats, and other creatures by cutting down on the amount of food given. The explanation for the result is simple; less food means fewer digestive enzymes are required, which contributes to a higher enzyme potential, which keeps death away as well as arming the body against disease.

There is an equally prolific scientific periodical literature reporting decrease in the activity of a number of enzymes in old age. Drs. Bartos and Groh, Charles University, Prague, Czechoslovakia, enlisted 10 young men and 10 men who were aged but healthy as experimental subjects and used a drug on all 20 men to stimulate the pancreatic juice flow. The juice was then pumped out and tested. It was found that the enzyme amylase was much weaker in the older men. Drs. Bartos, Groh, and others concluded that the enzyme deficiency of the older group was due to exhaustion in the cells of the pancreas. The real cause: the exhaustion of the enzyme potential of the many billions of cells of the whole organism, which, as we will see, are depleted toward the end of life by the unnatural needs of the body's digestive juices. In only rare cases has a weakened pancreatic secretion been proven to be caused by a defect in the pancreas. It should be obvious that the pancreas, which in the average American weighs 85 to 90 grams, or about 3 ounces, cannot begin to supply the vast amount of enzyme activity required by the pancreatic secretion, not to mention the tremendous need for protein to equip the enzyme complex. The pancreas must steal, beg, and borrow these entities stored in the whole body to make the enzyme complex. This is such an important point I have devoted an entire section to it later on. And I will show that the pancreas as well as the entire body is much the worse due to the acts of piracy upon the enzyme potential which must also try to furnish an adequate supply of metabolic enzymes.

There is some further evidence that can be interpreted to indicate the intimate connection between metabolic enzymes and the phenomenon we call life. In fact we are left with no escape from the realization that enzyme activity and the spark used to trigger all of our daily actions are one and the same. For instance, thinking involves enzyme activity. The man who first crystallized the protein of the enzyme complex, which carries the enzyme's biological activity factor, was Nobel laureate James B. Sumner of Cornell University. Sumner defined life as an orderly functioning of enzymes. I like to think of life as an integration of enzyme reactions. Life ends when the worn-out metabolic enzyme activity of the body machine drops to such a low point that it is unable to carry on vital enzyme reactions. This is the true trademark of old age. Old age and debilitated metabolic enzyme activity are synonymous. If we postpone the debilitation of metabolic enzyme activity, what we now call old age could become the glorious prime of life.

Consider the following research results. Burge and Burge, University of Illinois, attributed respiratory metabolism or oxidation to tissue catalase and measured this enzyme in the whole macerated bodies of Colorado potato beetles. They established values of 1750 units for young adult beetles, but only 900 units for older beetles.

Another researcher, Bodine of the University of Pennsylvania, likewise found that the catalase content in adult grasshoppers, potato beetles, and fireflies decreased with increasing old age. Sekla, Charles University, Prague, Czechoslovakia, showed that extracts of the whole bodies of older fruit flies contained less enzyme activity than did flies in the prime of life. The enzyme esterase, which performs digestive functions in the digestive tract and metabolic activities in the tissues, was tested. Lipase (an enzyme which dissolves fat) was measured in extracts of whole macerated rats by Falk, Noyes and Suguira. Compared to adult rats in their prime, the enzyme activity of this tissue enzyme was low in old rats. We can learn from this research that if you have young enzymes at age 80 you should be in the prime of life—not old. If you take in enzyme reinforcements during the younger years, your enzymes at 80 will be more like those at 40.

At the Israel Institute of Technology, nematodes (a type of worm) were chosen as a favorable organism for a study of aging, by Erlanger and Gershon. It was shown that in this tiny worm, three metabolic and digestive enzymes lost their pep when the animals became old. There are hundreds of metabolic enzymes, but considering the labor involved, we had better be grateful when someone is gracious enough to test even one of them. In the Israeli research the enzymes tested were choline esterase (nervous system), a-amylase (digestive system), and malic dehydrogenase (respiratory system).

In the Michael Reese Hospital, Chicago, the digestive enzymes of 93 human subjects, ranging in age from 12 to 96 years, were examined by Meyer, Spier, and Neuwelt in the 1930s and 1940s. Although the activity of these digestive enzymes is speeded and assisted by donor enzyme activity during the younger years, they also suffer the fate which is the price of squandering the enzyme potential over many years. The Michael Reese investigation discovered that the important digestive enzymes pepsin and trypsin were decreased in the old group to one-fourth of the strength of these same enzymes in the younger group. The amylase of the saliva was also markedly decreased in the old subjects, and the amylase and lipase of the pancreatic juice showed up slightly decreased in the aged.

FOOD ENZYMES ADD LIFE

The foregoing evidence clearly indicates the existence of a fixed enzyme potential in all living creatures. This potential, as I have shown, diminishes in time, subject to the conditions and pace of life. Humans eating an enzymeless diet use up a tremendous amount of their enzyme potential in lavish secretions of the pancreas and other digestive organs. The result is a shortened lifespan (65 years or less as compared with 100 or more), illness, and lowered resistance to stresses of all types, psychological and environmental. By eating foods with their enzymes intact and by supplementing cooked foods with enzyme capsules, we can stop abnormal and pathological aging processes. As a consequence of the improvements in health on such a regime, symptoms are alleviated and the response of the bodily immune system is strengthened.

Now let us turn to the mysterious life of the enzyme itself, its functions in the body, and its role in nutrition and health.

3

The Private Lives of Enzymes

THE SIGNIFICANCE OF ENZYMES IN FOOD AND HEALTH

We can close our minds and think of nutrition, with all of the knowledge gained about vitamins and minerals, as a completed science. But the fact remains that every ingredient in food must be accounted for, including the hundreds of food enzymes that comprise a distinct category of food elements. Food enzymes have been influencing the digestion and metabolism of living organisms for millions of years; modern man cannot forever ignore them. To better understand the role of enzymes, their basic anatomy and function in the human body and in the food we eat, this chapter will discuss many of the different enzymes found in modern and traditional foods, and their role in digestion and health. As you will see, the traditional use of enzyme-rich fermented foods and raw (versus cooked and pasteurized) dairy and other foods by "primitive" cultures is grounded in scientific fact, and is one of the important reasons for their vitality and relative freedom from degenerative diseases.

Enzymes and Life

One of the first scientists to announce a modified vitalistic view of the nature of the enzyme complex was Dr. L.T. Troland of Harvard University. In 1916 he wrote a paper entitled "The Enzyme Theory of Life" for a medical journal, in which he said: "The essence of life is catalysis. Life is something which has been built up about the enzyme; it is a corollary of enzyme activity." In 1921 Thomas Edison spoke of "the real units of life, consisting of millions of small entities living in the visible cells." In their book on enzymes published in 1958, the authorities Dixon and Webb, University of Cambridge, stated: "The whole subject of the origin of enzymes, like that of the origin of life, which is essentially the same thing, bristles with difficulties. We may surely say of the advent of enzymes, as Hopkins said of the advent of life, that it was the most improbable and the most significant event in the history of the universe."

When Professor Sumner, who received a Nobel Prize for his effort, first showed that enzymes could be crystallized, it was hailed in the press as the ultimate triumph in the solution of the enzyme riddle, an establishment of the enzyme's pedigree. But it is no such thing. We know no more about what actually makes enzymes tick than we knew before. If you take the suit off a man, the world may get a better view of what he really looks like. If all other clothing is removed, down to the naked body, still more light is shed on his appearance. But it does not tell us what goes on inside and what he is really like. Neither can we see what goes on inside of an enzyme crystal by viewing its naked exterior. The crystal discovery has been blown out of all proportion to its real worth in terms of fundamental physiology. It masks the true identity of the enzyme. Having a poignant bearing on these speculations is the observation of Dr. W.P. Jencks, Brandeis University, before a joint meeting of the Biochemical and Chemical Societies in Oxford in 1970: "You can define the anatomy of an enzyme without understanding its physiology."

Dr. K.F. Schaffner, University of Chicago, wrote in 1967: "Distinguished biologists and physicists have argued in the past, as well as quite recently, that it is impossible at the present time to explain the behavior of living organisms on the basis of their chemical constitution." In a paper entitled "Pre-Cell Evolution and the Origin of Enzymes," Simon Black of the National Institute of Health suggested in 1970 that processes now completed with enzymes in milliseconds may have once required hundreds of years. A.I. Oparin, Bach Institute of Biochemistry, Moscow, in a 1965 paper entitled "The Origin of Life and the Origin of Enzymes" stated: "The primary appearance of enzymes was inseparably connected with the appearance of life. We cannot repeat the process in the same way as it occurred in nature since it required billions of years to take place."

The Vitality Factor

Enzymes are substances that make life possible. They are needed for every chemical reaction that takes place in the human body. No mineral, vitamin, or hormone can do any work without enzymes. Our bodies, all of our organs, tissues, and cells, are run by metabolic enzymes. They are the manual workers that build our body from proteins, carbohydrates, and fats, just as construction workers build our homes. You may have all the raw materials with which to build, but without the workers (enzymes) you cannot even begin.

THE FUNCTIONS OF ENZYMES IN THE BODY

In 1966, the editor of *Scottish Medical Journal* editorialized in these words: "Probably nearly half of our daily production of protein in the body consists of enzymes. Indeed each of us, as with all living organisms, could be regarded as an orderly integrated succession of enzyme reactions." What this means is that our breathing, sleeping, eating, working, and even thinking are enzyme-dependent. The pancreas is the biggest factory devoted to turning out digestive enzymes. But it does not make enzymes any more than the United States Steel Corporation makes steel. Iron is shipped in and transformed into finished products. Similarly, the pancreas receives enzyme precursors from body cells or the bloodstream and supplies the finishing touches. The living body is under a great daily burden to produce the volume of enzymes necessary to run efficiently. Unfortunately we are not conscious of this, or we would be extremely concerned about how enzymes are dispensed, and be less likely to waste them. Enzymes are continually being used and eliminated in the urine, feces, and sweat. The laboratory in every hospital can find them there. They are needed in digesting food, running the heart, kidneys, liver, and lungs, and even in thinking.

Life could not exist without enzymes. Enzymes convert the food we eat into chemical structures that can pass through the cell membranes of the cells lining the digestive tract and into the bloodstream. Food must be digested so that it can ultimately pass through cell membranes. Enzymes also aid in converting the prepared food into new muscle, flesh, bone, nerves, and glands. Working with the liver they help store excess food for future energy and building needs.

They also assist the kidneys, lungs, liver, skin, and colon in their important eliminative tasks. Perhaps it would be easier to write about what enzymes don't do, for they are involved in almost every aspect of life!

One enzyme helps to build phosphorus into bone. Another causes blood to coagulate, stopping bleeding. Iron is bound in the red blood cells by another enzyme, while others provide oxidation—the union of oxygen with other substances. As the true alchemists of the body, enzymes can convert protein into fat, or sugar or carbohydrate into fat. Cooked carbohydrate food is used to fatten farm animals. Conversely, during an animal's long winter hibernation or a person's self-imposed fast for weight loss, enzymes convert fats to carbohydrates for energy. Although the following discussion will focus on enzymes in the digestive tract, it is important to keep in mind that enzymes perform thousands of metabolic tasks continuously.

Digestive Enzymes

The two most potent digestive enzymes secreted by the human body are amylase and protease. These deal with the digestion of two classes of foodstuffs, carbohydrates and proteins, respectively. Saliva supplies a high concentration of amylase, while stomach juice contains protease. The pancreas secretes digestive juices that contain both amylase and protease in high concentrations, along with a third enzyme, lipase, which deals with fats. Lipase, however, is present in a weaker concentration than amylase and protease. One other enzyme, maltase, which reduces maltose to dextrose, is secreted to a lesser extent by the pancreas. Further along the digestive tract, intestinal enzymes continue work on the partially digested foods.

Even though only amylase and protease are found in high concentrations in digestive juices, it would be incorrect to say that 2 enzymes do the majority of the work of digestion. This would fail to take account of food enzymes and some other enzymes present during digestion.

These food enzyme workers aren't lazy. They work day and night to build up and later break down the millions of cells in both plants and animals. For centuries humans have put these enzymes to work at predigesting foods before eating them. Fermented foods and aged foods are predigested by their own inherent enzymes or by starters such as those often used in the production of sourdough bread, yogurt, and some cheeses. Later in this chapter we will discuss in detail the traditional uses of enzymes in food preparation. For now, let's touch on some common foods and their food enzymes.

All uncooked foods contain an abundance of food enzymes which correspond to the nutritional highlights of the food. For example, dairy foods, oils, seeds, and nuts, which are relatively high in fat content, also contain relatively higher concentrations of the enzyme lipase which aids in the digestion of their fats. Carbohydrates, such as grains, contain higher concentrations of amylase and lesser amounts of lipase and protease. Lean meats, on the other hand, contain sizable amounts of protease in the form of cathepsin and little amylase. Low-calorie fruits and vegetables contain lesser amounts of protein and starch digestants and sizable quantities of the enzyme cellulase, which is needed to break down plant fibers. We could continue the list indefinitely, but the point is that nature has enclosed all raw foods with the correct and balanced amounts of food enzymes either for human consumption or eventual decomposition outside the human body.

Table 3.1 presents the results of investigations of various enzymes examined in the foods indicated. Obviously, other enzymes not listed are also present. This is a compendium of the reports to be found in the periodical literature.

Table 3.1
ENZYMES IN FOODS

Material	Authority	Year	Enzymes
Apple	M. Lieberman et al.	1966	Peroxidase
Banana	K. Kondo et al.	1928	Amylase, maltase, sucrase
Cabbage	B. Rubin et al.	1935	Amylase
Corn	V. N. Padwardhan et al.	1929	Amylase
Egg	H. Lineweaver et al.	1948	Tributyrinase, lipase phosphatase, peptidase, peroxidase, catalase, oxidase, amylase
Grape	A.T. Markh et al.	1957	Peroxidase, polyphenol-oxidase, catalase
Kidney bean	J. Labarre et al.	1946	Amylase, protease
Mango	A. K. Matto et al.	1968	Peroxidase, catalase phosphatase, dehydrogenase

Table 3.1, *Continued*

ENZYMES IN FOODS

Material	Authority	Year	Enzymes
Maple sap	E. Bois et al.	1938	Amylase
Meat	M. B. Berman	1967	Cathepsin
Meat	A.J. Lutalo-Bosa et al.	1969	Cathepsin
Milk	K.G. Weckel	1938	Catalase, galactase, lactase, amylase, oleinase, peroxidase, dehydrogenase, phosphatase
Mushroom	M.E. Dodonowa et. al.	1930	Maltase, glycogenase, amylase, protease, catalase
Potato	R. Pressey	1968	Invertase
Raw Honey	C.C. Gillette	1931	Catalase
Raw Honey	R.E. Lothrop et al.	1931	Amylase
Rice	D.V. Karmarker et al.	1931	Amylase
Soybean	N.V. Novotelnov	1935	Oxidase, protease, urease
Strawberry	I. Reifer et al.	1968	Dehydrogenase
Sugar cane	C.E. Hartt	1934	Amylase, catalase, ereptase invertase, maltase, oxidase, peroxidase, peptase, saccharase, tryosinase
Sweet potato	K.V. Giri	1934	Amylase
Tomato	H. Naito et al.	1938	Oxidase
Wheat	D.V. Karmarker et al.	1930	Amylase
Wheat	J.D. Mounfield	1938	Protease

OUR FIRST INTRODUCTION TO FOOD ENZYMES

From time immemorial, human babies have received dozens of enzymes from their mother's breast during the first years of their life. Some groups, such as the Eskimos, commonly nurse their young two or three years. Within the past century, however, many women have stopped nursing babies, feeding them pasteurized milk instead. Many babies get no milk enzymes now. Is this bad? The enzyme factory of the infant is thrown into high gear the very day it is born. Who can say what the effect will be fifty years hence? Or what will be carried over to pester the health of future generations? Considering the present ills of mankind it would be the height of folly for us to close our eyes to hidden, but very real, causes of disease. Only by opening our eyes can genuine progress ever be made in getting to the roots of our deadly cancer-and-heart-trouble kinds of ailments.

Dr. I.A. Arshavskii, a pediatrician, wrote a medical report in 1940 entitled "Lipase of Mother's Milk and Its Importance in Regard to the Disadvantages of Bottle Feeding." He was concerned about the fact that, whereas human milk has a good amount of lipase enzyme, when a baby sucks pasteurized milk from a bottle it gets almost none. Arshavskii believed that the lipase in human milk compensates for a deficiency in the pancreatic juice of the human infant and proposed the use of a lipase supplement in bottle feeding. The good doctor therefore is on record as a proponent of the thesis that food enzymes are useful in human nutrition.

On the other hand, today's mother, living the cola-drink kind of life, may not be able to supply milk as good as pasteurized milk. But a number of reports in the old medical literature, before soft drinks were so popular, attest to the superiority of breast feeding over bottle feeding. One of these, "Breast and Artificial Feeding," in the *Journal of the American Medical Association* for September, 1934, by Grulee, Sanford and Herron of Rush Medical College, involved 20,061 babies. There were three categories: 48.5 percent were entirely breast-fed, 43.0 percent were partially breast-fed, and 8.5 percent had pasteurized cow's milk. The figures for morbidity (sickness) are given in Table 3.2.

Table 3.2
MORBIDITY OF BREAST-FED AND BOTTLE-FED BABIES

	Breast-fed	Partially Breast-fed	Bottle-fed
Morbidity (20,061 subjects)	37.4 %	53.8 %	63.6%

Adapted from C.G. Grulee et al., "Breast and Artificial Feeding," *Journal of the American Medical Association*, 103(10):735, September, 1934.

It can be seen from the above table that the babies who were entirely breast-fed (receiving a full quota of milk enzymes) had far less sickness than babies who were only partially breast-fed or who were bottle-fed. It can be pointed out that these latter two groups had either a smaller intake of food enzymes or none at all. If anyone believes the differences as revealed by the figures in the table can be accounted for in some other way than on the basis of the food enzyme intake, they are at liberty to point out specifically the details.

I do not intend to devote much space to the concept that immunity factors may pass from the mother to her nursing infant, because informed people already know or suspect it. But few are aware that both human and bovine milk have scores of enzymes. The enzymes in bovine milk are destroyed by pasteurization. I wish to supply enough information to give readers a choice of how much weight to assign each possible contributing factor in a given case of infant sickness or death. Shahani et al., in "Enzymes in Bovine Milk," *Journal of Dairy Science* 56:531-43 (1973) stated that at least 20 enzymes have been either purified or isolated in cow's milk. The investigators confess that the function of most of these enzymes is not known after they are swallowed as food. It would be naive to assume that so many enzymes in a single food could be taken into the body of an infant (digestive fluids are poorly established in babies) and not exert an influence in some functions. I prefer to emphasize the fact that there are many enzymes in milk, that they are largely destroyed by pasteurization, and then let people make up their minds whether or not these enzymes are favorable to health and protection against disease.

Even when nursing at the breast, babies did not gain immunity from many diseases from their mothers. But they did get milk enzymes. Whether a lack of any of these enzymes in pasteurized bovine milk contributes toward infant morbidity or mortality has not been established. But there are records of doctors calling for amylase supplementation in bottle feeding because human milk is rich in amylase, while bovine milk, even when unpasteurized, is quite poor in this enzyme. The infant's salivary glands do not secrete amylase at an early age, and this enzyme is needed when starchy food is eaten. Pancreatic lipase is another enzyme called for by doctors, because the infant's pancreatic secretions are not well established, and commercial milk has little lipase.

Milk is the only food young animals receive for many months after birth. They grow on it, ingesting a large assortment of milk enzymes, and are healthy. That should prove, better than any laboratory test, that it is a complete food, at least for a nursing baby or animal. The adequacy of the nutrition secured from the mammary gland is confirmed by the fact that feeding at the breast has been practiced for about 200 million years. Milk from the cow contains the following major enzymes according to a report supplied in 1938 by K.G. Weckel, University of Wisconsin: catalase, galactase, lactase, amylase, oleinase, peroxidase, dehydrogenase, and phosphatase. Phosphatase is an enzyme that has been used by health departments to make sure that the temperature used in pasteurization was high enough to destroy bacteria. For example, if milk was pasteurized at 145° F for a half-hour, it would not only kill the bacteria but also kill nearly all of the phosphatase and other enzymes. If more than a small amount of phosphatase is found in the milk, it will not pass the "Phosphatase Test."

ENZYMES, GRAINS, AND GERMINATION

Grains such as wheat, barley, corn, and rice are used extensively, but knowledge of their food enzymes is less widespread. In the grain family more is known about barley enzymes because barley is a staple in the brewing industry. Barley is germinated (sprouted) by the malting process, in which the enzymes, particularly amylase, increase.

Any seed can be made to germinate by increasing its moisture and holding it at the proper temperature. Resting seeds contain starch, which is a storage product and a source of future energy when conditions become ideal for the seed to germinate and grow into a plant. In nature, seeds sometimes must rest or hibernate for months or years before conditions become satisfactory for them to grow. Enzymes are present in the resting seed but are prevented from being active by the presence of enzyme inhibitors. Germination neutralizes the inhibitors and releases the enzymes. Enzyme inhibitors are part of the seed machinery and serve a purpose. But these inhibitors are out of place in our bodies. They could stop our enzymes from working. Ways to get rid of enzyme inhibitors will be explained in Chapter 7.

Germination greatly increases the enzyme action. At the proper time in either natural or artifical germination, the enzyme amylase turns the starch into sugar which can circulate freely in the growing plant and act as a source of energy. The same process takes place when we eat starchy cereals or potatoes. Ptyalin is the name for the amylase type of enzyme in our saliva that starts converting the starch into sugar. Starch molecules cannot mix with our blood and circulate around the body, but sugar gets around to every nook and cranny of the body to deliver energy.

In malted barley, the enzymes make the sugar known as maltose, which is processed into beer. Although it is possible to multiply the enzymes of corn and wheat by germination, there is little market for these products. But in the Orient, rice is modified by enzymes to produce the alcoholic beverage sake. Enzymes have been utilized to produce Oriental foods for centuries. Various soybean products, such as miso, tofu, and tempeh, depend on enzymes for proper conversion to good foods. These have supplied a substantial part of the food needs of Asiatics for thousands of years, and are becoming increasingly popular in the West.

Modern Grain Is Low in Enzymes

As related to digestion in the animal body, the principal enzymes in grains are amylase, protease, and lipase. When fed to farm animals these grain enzymes initiate starch, protein, and fat digestion in the upper part of the digestive tract and even continue it in the cecum (the beginning of the large intestine) in some instances. Before the advent of factory farms, grain was partially germinated, but modern grain consists of dormant (resting) seeds. Because combine-harvested grains have a decreased enzyme content, their nutrient constituents may not be so readily digestible by livestock and poultry as in former times, accounting for the increasingly common practice of adding enzymes to the feed. The use of the modern combine, while tremendously decreasing the work of the farmer, has made it necessary to add the enzymes amylase and protease to white flour to make a loaf of bread uniform in size and texture. Needless to say, the human consumer gets no benefit from the enzyme addition because baking kills these delicate benefactors. In former times grain was harvested and sheaved. The sheaves were put into shocks and allowed to stand in the field for several weeks. Then the shocks were gathered and built into stacks which stood in the field for several more weeks before threshing. During this period of weathering in the field the grain seeds were exposed to rain and dew which soaked into the sheaves. The grain could pick up this moisture, and, with heat from the sun, conditions were ideal for favoring a degree of germination and enzyme multiplication in the grain. The modern combine harvester removes the grain from the stalk immediately after cutting and permits it to be hauled away to the granary. Hence there is no weathering and consequent enzyme development, resulting in a mature but dormant seed.

We can see that those in the malting and brewing industries have been interested in using enzymes, but only for helping in producing their products. Millers of flour and bakers also like enzymes, but here again, just to serve their own ends. Similarly, when feeders of livestock and poultry add enzymes to the feed, they are interested only in the profit. In none of these instances does the consumer get any enzyme benefit from these efforts. All of the enzymes are destroyed in the kitchen or the food-torturing equipment in the factories. The same holds true in the meat packing and processing industry. There are a number of enzymes in meat, but, as we will see, they are all destroyed before they reach the consumer.

TENDERIZING ENZYMES

The aging of meat and game to promote its tenderness and enhance its flavor has been practiced for a long time. The aging process consists of keeping the product at the proper environment of moisture and temperature. This allows the enzyme cathepsin within the tissues to slowly digest the hung meat by a process not unlike that which occurs in the digestive tract and which is known as autolysis. This is a good example of the operation of food enzymes. In those carnivores swallowing an entire animal, the catheptic enzymes of the prey become food enzymes and act the same way in the stomach of the host as they do when aging meat. Sprinkling tenderizers on meat is now practiced extensively. These powders commonly contain an enzyme extracted from unripe papaya or from fungi. The powdered enzymes work better if they are stirred in warm water and applied to the meat after perforating it with a fork. In this manner the enzyme can penetrate deeper, which improves tenderness. It is well to wait before cooking to allow some time for the enzyme to act, but not too long because the final product might become too soft. Here again the consumer gets no benefit from the enzyme cathepsin and other meat enzymes which carnivorous animals consume in their food, since these enzymes are destroyed in cooking. Neither does he profit from the tenderizing enzyme. They all perish in the throes of heat treatment in the kitchen. One practice of the meat processing industry is tenderizing meat on the hoof by injecting enzymes into the circulatory system of the live animal shortly before slaughter. The enzymes are carried around the body by the circulating blood, permeating the interior parts of the flesh, and are believed to function more effectively than when applied to the surface of meats.

THIS IS PREDIGESTION—RAW HONEY

Raw honey is noteworthy for having considerable plant amylase. The amylase does not come from the bee but is a true plant enzyme, concentrated from the pollen of flowers. Its origin was established when it was shown by Vansell that the optimal pH for activity was around 4 for plant amylase, and near 7 for bee amylase. If you wish to predigest a starchy food such as bread, spread some raw honey on it. The moment the honey and bread come into contact, the honey enzyme starts predigestion, and as you chew, more digestion takes place. If the bread with its honey-enzyme coating is allowed to stand at room temperature for 15 minutes before you eat it, there will be less work for salivary amylase.*

The amylase from raw honey readily converts starch into maltose sugar, but ordinary heated liquid honey will have no effect. Commercial honey is heated upwards of 24 hours to prevent it from turning hard and opaque. Heating destroys the amylase which is richer in raw honey than in most other foods. The German Honey Ordinance of 1930 ordered that honey was not to be sold for table use unless it contained the enzyme amylase. All other honey was to be used by the bakery trade. The Netherlands passed a law in 1925 stating that amylase must be present in honey unless it is labeled heated honey. In the United States, however, there is no requirement preventing honey from being deprived of its enzyme content. In 1931, R.E. Lothrop and H.S. Paine, of the Bureau of Chemistry and Soils, Washington, D.C., investigated the amylase content of 26 types of American honey. Their results support the conclusion that it is truly a plant food enzyme.

The reason bees make honey is to use it for food during the colder months when there are no blooms from which to extract nectar. The beekeeper wishes to maintain a profitable operation. So he takes away more honey than he should. The result is that long before spring vegetation comes to life the bees have eaten their winter food supply. At this point the beekeeper puts out trays of sugar dissolved in water and the bees feed on it. This practice of feeding sugar to bees is rather universal in northern countries, and it cannot be in the best interest of consumers, who later eat the honey produced by bees who were forced to subsist upon such a skeletonized article as refined sugar. No scientist working with animals in a laboratory would dream of feeding them only sugar! But it does increase profits. During World War II there was a sugar shortage and sugar rationing. But honey producers got a special high priority rating for withdrawing thousands of tons of sugar for feeding bees.

---

*Publisher's Note: Recent research has shown that honey, whether raw or pasteurized, should not be fed to infants who are under one year of age. Spores in the honey may cause infant botulism, an uncommon but potentially fatal disease.

RAW DAIRY FOODS

Under the anti-ecological modern conditions of life, there is some justification for tolerating the pasteurization of milk because raw milk can become contaminated while being handled on its way to the consumer. Raw milk is a convenient vehicle for the transmission of communicable disease. The need for pasteurization is abolished on a family farm where milk is produced only for its members. As a small boy I used to spend my school vacation on a farm where the animals received no food except that which they could find in the pasture and woods. These were not heavy milk producers with enormous udders. The cows were never ill; the need for a veterinarian was negligible. Contrast this with championship milkers with their large udders which are usually afflicted with mastitis and its associated discharge of pus. This unsavory condition usually requires almost continuous use of penicillin to keep the milk flowing. These champions are fed objectionable concentrates and other materials at odds with Enzyme Nutrition. What will you have, less good milk, or an abundance of milk incriminated as a cause of heart and artery disease?

For 12 years Russian researchers have been observing 180 men and women living in and around the town of Dageston, and ranging in age from 90 to 100 years. The men and women living in town were heavier in weight and had more disease of blood vessels than the people living in the nearby mountains. All of the people studied ate some meat, but the town dwellers ate more carbohydrate food than the mountain folk, whose diet was mainly dairy products and vegetable foods. Modern nutrition condemns butter as a source of cholesterol, but these Russians managed to reach ages past 90 while eating butter freely. (Voprosy Pitaniya 32:46-50, 1973.) In another study, Metchnikoff studied communities of Bulgarians who ate mainly raw dairy food—and lived past 100. Are we to close our eyes to this evidence? Perhaps there is a difference between the milk and butter of these simple people and ours. In fact, more than 90 percent of the enzymes in milk are destroyed by pasteurization. Chemists have identified 35 separate enzymes in raw milk, with lipase one of the chief enzyme actors. How much longer are we to ignore the value of food enzymes?

Unpasteurized milk and butter were used for thousands of years, with a history of conferring good health on their users. Since the time of Hippocrates, physicians used raw milk and raw butter as therapeutic agents to treat disease. Whole nations formerly depended upon dairy products as major sources of food. But when pasteurization was introduced, dairy products strangely and precipitously lost their health charms, almost as if somebody waved an evil wand and presto, dairy products were instantly cursed. For example, in the days before milk and butter lost their lipase due to the heat of pasteurization, millions of people lived on dairy products without getting atherosclerosis (clogged arteries due to cholesterol deposits) because lipase knows how to handle cholesterol.

We have lost our ability to tame this killer. Lipase was also a valued guest in olive oil and other oils when they were thick and opaque, but had to give up its residence when the factories made them clear. The commercial production of these oils coincides with the rise of cancer-related deaths in modern society. These strong indications of the value of lipase offer reasons why lipase should be given high priority in research to test its capacity to neutralize pathogenic effects.

THE ESKIMO AND A RAW DIET

It is important that we put the spotlight on the primitive, isolated Eskimo. Since the airplane has invaded the far north, this hardy and healthy people have largely accepted some of the evil ways of civilization. But the original habits and customs of the Eskimo can give us valuable insights on how to achieve a high level of health: he practiced conservation of body enzymes by arranging for outside enzymes to help digest his food.

I am not suggesting that you emulate the primitive Eskimo and try living on raw meat. Plant food is virtually nonexistent in the far north. The Eskimo had to adapt to what was available and was forced to modify animal flesh in ways to serve not only as fuel but to maintain excellent health and prevent disease. There is no evidence that humans can live on a diet containing large quantities of unmodified fresh raw meat. Carnivores prefer some of their meat partially autolyzed and contrive to have what they eat exposed to a maximum degree of digestion by the proteolytic enzyme cathepsin. The Eskimo always uses the food enzyme cathepsin of meat and fish to help both its predigestion and digestion. In the following paragraphs, I will summarize the observations of some authorities on the life of the primitive Eskimo. Their observations illustrate the appropriateness of the word "Eskimo," which is derived from an American Indian language, and means "he eats it raw."

What Authorities Say About the Eskimo Diet

D.B. MacMillan, an explorer and authority on the Arctic who lived 6 years with primitive Eskimos in Greenland, stated in *National Geographic*: "Holding a piece of raw, frozen liver in one hand, and a piece of seal blubber in the other, they sat down to feast, the bread and butter of the Eskimo. After a walrus hunt, they have a dinner of raw clams eaten right out of the stomach of the walrus."

K. Birket-Smith in his book *The Eskimo* noted that meat is stored to undergo autolysis, which produces new flavors so that "walrus meat tastes like old, sharp and rich cheese."

W.O. Douglas wrote in *National Geographic*, May 1964, "The Banks Island Eskimos said that frozen fish and frozen caribou seem to provide more 'strength' than cooked food."

In Robert A. Bartlett's book *The Last Voyage of the Karluk*, Small Maynard & Co., publishers (1916), he described a meal with Siberian Eskimos of raw, frozen reindeer as good eating.

C.M. Garber, in *Eating With the Eskimos*, Hygeia 16:242 (1938) said, "Alaskan Eskimos are heavy eaters of lean meats and large amounts of blubber. In only a few instances did they cook their food. The usual and customary method was to devour it raw." Accoridng to Garber, the Eskimos thrive on *titmuck*, which is frozen, raw fish, reduced to a consistency requiring it to be ladled.

Bishop J.L. Coudert of the Yukon traveled by dog team among his Indian camps for 20 years, living on a diet composed almost solely of moose meat and fish, frozen and eaten raw. In a press clipping, Bishop Coudert said "I feel better every year."

Dr. W.A. Thomas, physician with a polar expedition to Greenland, wrote: "The diet of the Greenland Eskimo includes the meat of whale, walrus, seal, caribou, musk ox, arctic hare, polar bear, fox, ptarmigan, birds and fish, all eaten usually and preferably raw."

Dr. I.M. Rabinowitch was a member of early Canadian expeditions to study the life, customs, and health of the Canadian Arctic Eskimo. He reported that meat was eaten raw and that the livers of practically all animals except the white bear were eaten. Meat was cached and eaten in an autolyzed state, and the contents of the stomachs of walrus and caribou were used.

The anthropologist V. Stefansson lived among the Eskimos of northern Canada for some 7 years and became an authority of primitive Eskimo life. His reports appeared in many journals where he emphasized the excellent state of their health and freedom from disease. Although the usual practice for venturers into the far north was to provision an expedition with salt pork and hardtack, Stefansson partook of the Eskimo diet. It required some time for him to get used to the practice of eating meat raw or half-cooked, to overcome his craving for salt, and still longer to learn to enjoy the flavor of smelly, high raw, frozen fish, and to experience the resulting feeling of well-being after eating it. Stefansson observed that the high fish was retrieved from the pit in which it had been buried (on top of the area of perpetual frost, the freezer of the Eskimos) and brought into the dwelling to melt. He described the consistency and appearance as that of ice cream. The partially digested plant food of the caribou stomach is removed, dressed with oil, and eaten as a salad. After returning from the Arctic, Stefansson placed himself under medical observation and study at Bellevue Hospital (Lieb, 1929), and no signs of deficiency diseases were found.

Dr. J.A. Urquhart makes some illuminating comments that should dispel the apprehension and fear of "ptomaine" poisoning that most people feel when they see the Eskimo eat so-called "high" meat and fish. Dr. Urquhart wrote: "They kill a caribou and allow it to lie for several days without disemboweling it or cutting it up. An interesting point in connection with high uncooked food is brought out by one's experience with dogs. If a dog team is worked hard daily for two weeks and fed with fresh fish caught under the ice and frozen without opportunity of becoming high, that team will lose weight and show definite signs of wear and tear. If the team is fed with hung or high fish, they will be as good at the end of that time as at the start, and often will have put on a little weight. The explanation is that it is probably more of an autolysis than a bacterial decomposition, or, in other words, pre-digestion."

Let us have Dr. Rabinowitch continue the dialogue about "high" meat and fish: "As in man, no ill effects have been observed in the dog because of the eating of putrefied meats. The average concentration of non-protein nitrogenous constitutents of the bloods of 46 Eskimos was found to be higher than of peoples elsewhere, apparently due to the enormous quantities of meats eaten. Meat is eaten in a putrefied state. This, it would appear, is the explanation of the high amino acid value (proteolysis)."

Let us not lose sight of the fact that meat and fish have widespread and ample stores of the proteolytic enzyme cathepsin that is always ready to get busy and dismantle its owner's dead body when conditions are right. These food sources are also equipped with the enzyme lipase, which craves a workout on fat. The work that these enzymes do to implement and supplement digestion may be far more important than merely accounting for the high values of non-protein nitrogen and amino acids showing up in Dr. Rabinowitch's tests. Their influence is more profound. According to the law of Adaptive Secretion of Digestive Enzymes, organisms eating these partly digested "high" foods will need to secrete fewer enzymes. And the energy so saved may well be the very ingredient explaining the stamina and high energy levels experienced by Eskimos and other peoples on these rations.

The secret of the good health of the carnivorous Eskimo is not that he eats meat, but that he forbids his personal enzymes to digest all of it. We can do the same with proteins, carbohydrates, and fats from plant foods.

PREDIGESTED FOODS IN OTHER CULTURES

As we have seen, the practice of eating autolyzed (predigested) meat and fish has been reported by a number of authorites as being common among diverse groups of Eskimos scattered over the northern regions and not related to each other. These groups are willing to overlook the objectionable odor because experience has taught them that the partially digested food gives them more endurance. Other groups of people around the world have likewise shared in finding unique values in partially digested protein food, such as aged cheese and hung, aged meat. In other words, autolyzed food, which has already been broken down into peptones and proteoses, uses less of our personal enzymes. This is what produces the feeling of well-being and surplus energy.

Epicures among us can forgive the strong odor of some cheeses or of hung, aged meats, to gain the flavor and added benefits of protease enzymatic wizardry. The instinct of saving endogenous enzymes extends from the frozen Arctic to the steaming jungles. Once, when Pygmies were busily devouring the "ripe" carcass of an elephant dead several days in the heat of equatorial Africa they were asked why they ate such putrid food. One of them replied that they were eating the meat and not the odor.

I would not advocate very strongly the eating of raw flesh, since it may contribute to an increase in parasitic infections. Nevertheless, there are a number of traditional foods, predigested by enzyme processes, that are common in other cultures. Let us examine them briefly.

In the *National Geographic* (1970), William S. Ellis described *kibbeh*, the national dish of Lebanon. It consists basically of raw lamb and crushed wheat. These foods are pounded together for about an hour in a large stone mortar, then kneaded, seasoned, and eaten raw—*kibbeh niebeh*. The enzymes cathepsin and lipase of the lamb, and the protease, amylase, and lipase of wheat, being liberated from their bondage by pulverization, cooperate to achieve predigestion and inactivation of enzyme inhibitors during the hour the food is being pulverized. Thereafter the predigestion continues both before and after the food is eaten, until the stomach acidity becomes very strong. People who eat this Lebanese dish save their own enzymes.

Ernie Bradford tells about the highly prized *skerpikjot*—raw wind-cured mutton—in a 1970 issue of National Geographic. It was at one time a main ingredient of the diet in the Faeros Islands of the North Atlantic. Air-drying the meat in a slat-sided shed for a year or more gave ample time for the enzymes of the meat to convert the protein into the same materials the stomach and intestine produce when protein is eaten. The result was an uncooked delicacy with a pungent odor and a taste of high, cheesy mutton. Mr. Bradford learned to enjoy it and to appreciate what the Faeroese claim for it—"that it contains more energy than any other local food." These people could sense that it saved something quite precious for them.

During thousands of years, millions upon millions of Asiatic people have improved soybeans and other seeds for human food by exposing them to the action of enzymes in fungal plants, mainly of the aspergillus variety. These fungal enzymes promote predigestion of the protein, carbohydrate, and fat of the food during the preparation process, before it is eaten. This conserves the enzyme potential of the body and thereby fosters a longer lifespan. *Tofu kan, tofu p'i* and *yuba* are Chinese dishes resulting from food after being worked on by fungal enzymes. *Kabitofu* is a Chinese food prepared from soybean curd by the action of these enzymes. *Toyu* is a Philippine soy food, the result of the enzyme action. A vegetable cheese called *tofu* is made from soybean curd through the agency of fungal enzymes. *Natto* is a similar product. Miso is a soybean, rice or barley breakfast food improved by the enzyme action and used as a porridge in Japan. A soybean-enzyme food known as *tempeh* was used for centuries by the people of Java.

According to Lewis Cotlow in his book, *Amazon Head Hunters*, the Indians of the Amazon River basin have shown us how the human organism can best handle large amounts of starch with a great saving of endogenous enzymes: boiled yucca, which comes from a starchy tuber and supplies much food and drink for the people of the Amazon basin. The yucca drink is known as *nijimanche* among the Jivaros Indians. Cotlow states that it has a malty flavor, seems very nourishing, as much food as beverage—the staff of life for these people. The constant and endless task of some of the women is the making of nijimanche by chewing the yucca and expelling the thoroughly masticated product into large jars and allowing it to be digested by the amylase of saliva. Most adults drink 4 or 5 quarts a day.

Another clan on the Amazon River known as the Yagua have an equivalent for *nijimanche* which they call *masato*. The only difference is that they add some cane sap to the yucca mixture. The Colorado Indians of South America have a masticated *nijimanche* called *malakachisa* which also contains cane sap, giving it an apple-ciderish flavor. The starch used is not refined in any way and at the high equatorial temperatures, it is rapidly digested to a sugar stage ouside of the body, requiring only finishing touches by the consumer's personal enzymes.

Let's have an American equivalent of *nijimanche*. In technological societies such as our own, unrefined starchy foods could be masticated mechanically to take the place of chewing. There is a choice of several enzymes that could do everything performed by the saliva of the Indian women. To prevent the product from turning into alcohol, it could be refrigerated and delivered to consumers like milk. There is little doubt that consuming unrefined starch in this way would be a vast improvement over bread, crackers, potatoes, and cereals. The work would be done by enzymes in factories instead of by endogenous enzymes. Just think of the tremendous health benefits of using a combination enzyme food-beverage over empty cola drinks!

ENZYMES DIGEST THEIR OWN FOODS

Let us turn our attention to the extent to which the enzymes in food are capable of digesting their own ingredients. The banana is an excellent example. The banana has about 20 percent starch when green. The enzyme amylase changes the banana into 20 percent sugar when the fruit is kept in a warm temperature for a few days and becomes speckled. About one-quarter of this sugar is dextrose (glucose), needing no further digestion. The amylase in bananas works on banana starch, but not readily on other starches, for example, potato starch. The ripe banana contains high-class raw calories which have not earned the evil reputation of cooked calories. Ripe bananas will not make you fat. Let a fat person eat all the ripe bananas he wishes on an exclusive banana diet and see what happens. When banana enzymes have done their work there is that much less work for your enzymes to do. This is predigestion. By eating more raw calories and fewer cooked ones, you will get predigestion to work for you.

Banana enzymes efficiently convert starch into sugars in a short time. Likewise, after barley is germinated commercially by malting, its enzymes get stronger and are able to turn its starch into maltose (a type of sugar). You may read statements from time to time that outside enzymes from food or supplements are permanently inactivated or digested in the stomach after being swallowed. You may judge the worth of these remarks by consulting the evidence presented in Chapter 1.

I will discuss the use of dietary enzyme supplements at length in Chapter 6. For now, let us look at the role of exogenous food enzymes and endogenous digestive enzymes in light of two very important discoveries.

4

Two Important Discoveries

THE FOOD ENZYME STOMACH AND THE LAW OF ADAPTIVE SECRETION OF DIGESTIVE ENZYMES

The discovery of the food-enzyme stomach, which enables humans to predigest foods before they undergo more thorough digestion by the action of strong digestive juices secreted in the stomach and small intestine, and the discovery of the Law of Adaptive Secretion of Digestive Enzymes, which states that digestive enzymes are called upon according to the foods eaten, are keys to the Food Enzyme Concept. If the stomach is performing its proper role, and we are eating our foods uncooked, a large portion of the intake will be partially digested before reacting with the stronger digestive juices found there. Moreover, if uncooked food is eaten, fewer of your body's internal digestive enzymes will be called upon to perform the digestive function. That is, the body adapts to the plentiful supply of enzymes in the uncooked foods by secreting less of its own digestive enzymes— this preserves your internal enzyme supplies for the important work of maintaining metabolic harmony.

THE FOOD-ENZYME STOMACH

Predigestion by food enzymes occurs in every creature on earth. The only exception is the human being on an enzymeless diet. Many creatures are provided with a separate food-enzyme stomach. In primates and man the stomach has two parts with separate functions, the first part being the food-enzyme stomach. As we have seen, in large carnivores and snakes the stomach is often distended by food to such an extent that the entrance of stomach digestive juice, including pepsin, is prevented until the prey is more or less liquefied by its own digestive juices and the proteolytic cathepsin of its tissues. It appears that evolution has contrived adaptations and mechanisms to ensure that outside enzymes are forced to digest part of the food, and furthermore, that the law of Adaptive Secretion of Digestive Enzymes is also part of nature's plan to prevent enzyme waste by oversecretion. The predator inherits the protein, fat, vitamins, and minerals of the prey: it gets everything, including the prey's enzymes.

Current research supports the discovery of the human food-enzyme stomach. My research and physiology texts and hundreds of scientific papers have shown that peptic digestion of protein takes place in the lower part of the stomach. The upper part is where the enzymes in food, or enzymes taken with the food, participate in digestion. I have called this the food-enzyme stomach. Except in the cases of raw fermented and germinated foods, this is where initial predigestion occurs—the first step in the digestion of protein, fat, and starch by exogenous enzymes. (As you will recall, scientists term enzymes made by the body endogenous and those in food or digestive supplements, exogenous.)

The lower stomach performs the second step in predigestion, but of protein only. In the upper part of the small intestine the digestive juice of the pancreas continues the digestion of all the nutrients. But even this cannot be acknowledged to be complete digestion, but only an advanced phase of predigestion. Final digestion of food is accomplished by the cells lining the small intestine. Digestion in the food-enzyme stomach is no less important than digestion farther along in the alimentary canal.

The human stomach, like the stomach of a rat (see Figure 4.1), is relatively simple anatomically, and can be divided into sections with their own distinct functions. The illustration shows food eaten by a rat in three successive stages, the feed of each stage stained with a different color for identification purposes. After the contents settled in three layers (identified by the numerals 1, 2, and 3), the stomach was frozen and removed for examination. Number 1 was the first and largest feeding; number 2 and number 3 were subsequent smaller feedings, each feeding making a nest cradling the next one. The numerals also identify and point to the sections of the stomach; number 1, the pyloric section where pepsin and hydrochloric acid act to digest protein; and numbers 2 and 3, the fundic and cardiac sections—the

Figure 4.1

THREE LAYERS OF FOOD IN FROZEN STOMACH OF RAT

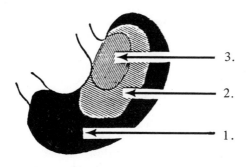

3.

2.

1.

Illustration by the German physiologist, Grutzner.

site where salivary and food enzymes function. This latter, the food-enzyme stomach, is the place where salivary and exogenous enzymes digest carbohydrates, proteins, and fats.

It may seem incredible in this enlightened age, but there is still controversy about the functioning of the stomach. I believe that the following data are the most accurate. The commonly held doctrines needing correction are: that the whole stomach is involved in a churning action which causes food as it is swallowed to be vigorously and almost instantly mixed with acid and pepsin; that the main job of the stomach is to digest protein and that very little starch is digested; that all digestion in the stomach is brought about by pepsin which requires strong acid, and that there is no gastric digestion with weaker acid; and that salivary enzymes, food enzymes, and supplementary enzymes are rapidly and permanently inactivated by gastric hydrochloric acid and are digested by pepsin.

The evidence presented clearly shows that the stomach is physiologically divided into an upper and a lower section. The upper section has no peristalsis, acid, or pepsin, so the food is not agitated or mixed with acid. At the tail end of the upper section some pepsin appears but it can do nothing until it mixes with the acid in the lower section. In the lower section the food is not churned, but just squeezed and pushed along. This arrangement allows ptyalin (amylase), food enzymes, and supplementary enzymes ample time to predigest starches,

Table 4.1
FACTS ABOUT THE STOMACH

Authority	Evidence
Gray's Anatomy	"It has apparently been demonstrated that the stomach con sists of two parts physiologically distinct. The cardiac portion of the stomach is a food reservoir in which salivary digestion continues; the pyloric portion is the seat of active gastric digestion. Cannon affirms that there are no peristaltic waves in the cardiac portion."
Cunningham's Anatomy	"The empty stomach is a contracted tubular organ, except at the fundus where it appears to be always dilated. When food is taken it runs down to the point where the gastric walls are in contact with one another. As the stomach becomes filled the whole of the body of the organ becomes dilated, but the fundus and cardiac portion more particularly so, and these two latter regions act as a storehouse."
Howell's Physiology	"The older view was that the contents of the stomach are kept in a general rotary movement so as to become more or less uniformly mixed; but Cannon's observations, and those of Grutzner, indicate that the material at the fundic end may remain undisturbed for a long time and thus escape mixture with the acid gastric juice, so far at least as the interior of the mass is concerned. This fact is of importance in connection with the salivary digestion of the starchy foods. There is every reason to believe, therefore, that salivary digestion may be carried on in the stomach to an important extent."
"The central cells furnish the digestive enzymes of the stomach—pepsin and rennin—and the parietal cells the hydrochloric acid. The parietal cells are massed in the glands of the middle of prepyloric region of the stomach, they are scanty in the fundus. The bulk of the food in the fundus becomes impregnated first with pepsin, then, as it slowly moves into the prepyloric region, the acid constituent is added."
R. Merten et al., University of Cologne, Germany	In addition to pepsin, gastric juice contains a catheptic protease. Tests on human subjects showed marked digestion by cathepsin in the stomach, the magnitude of which was at least as great as that shown by pepsin.

Table 4.1, *Continued*

FACTS ABOUT THE STOMACH

Authority	Evidence
J.M. Beazell, Department of Physiology, Northwestern University	"It is generally taught that the stomach is of little or no importance in starch digestion and, at least by implication, that it plays a relatively important role in the digestion of protein." Dr. Beazell tested digestion in 11 normal young male adult human subjects by feeding them a meal. The meal was removed from the stomach in one hour and examined. Of the food remaining in the stomach, 20 percent of the starch, and less than 3 percent of the protein had been digested. Dr. Beazell stated that "In view of these observations it is felt that the conventional concept that the stomach plays an unimportant role in the digestion of starch and an important role in the digestion of protein, is open to revision."
W.H. Taylor, Department of Clinical Biochemistry, University of Oxford	The gastric juice of 25 normal human subjects was investigated by Dr. Taylor. It was found to have two zones of maximal activity, in the area of pH 2 and pH 4, corresponding to the enzymes pepsin and cathepsin, respectively. Dr. Taylor stated: "Proteolysis at the maximum between pH 3.3 and 4.0 could be approximately as effective as that at pH 1.6–2.4."
G. Milhand et al., University of Geneva	In normal gastric juice the activity of pepsin and cathepsin is about equal.
E. Freudenberg, German Scientist	It was shown that the human stomach secretes pepsin and cathepsin. There are other reports in the literature about cathepsin which I do not feel it is necessary to introduce.
D. Maestrini	Starch protects salivary amylase from inactivation by gastric hydrochloric acid.
S. Pasrore	Starch acts as a buffer between hydrochloric acid and the enzyme of saliva.

proteins, and fats before they move into the lower section where food is acted upon by acid and pepsin.

The anatomist Cunningham, and the physiologist Howell, stoutly proclaim that the human stomach is actually two stomachs with two separate and distinct functions, each confined to either the upper or lower section. The lower section is stated to be constricted and flat when empty, while the upper section is open and has few, if any, glands to produce enzymes and acid and no peristaltic action, remaining quiescent at all times. The path of food can be traced in Figure 4.1. When food is swallowed, settling later into layer number 1, it first goes into the area marked by number 3. In this area, food is not churned or disturbed by peristalsis. After succeeding feedings, it overflows, opening and distending the flat and contracted pyloric area (number 1). In the prolonged intervening period, the food in the cardiac and fundic area—the food-enzyme stomach—has been undergoing carbohydrate, protein, and fat digestion by ptyalin and the amylase, protease, and lipase of exogenous (outside) enzymes for up to one hour. Because of the extremely low pH needed for peptic digestion, much time is needed for secretion of hydrochloric acid to lower the pH.

When the optimum pH for peptic activity is finally attained, the pepsin still cannot go into the food-enzyme stomach without moving against gravity—uphill, so to speak. You would have to stand on your head for a spell to permit pepsin to go into the food-enzyme stomach to do its work. But nature makes this unnecessary by giving the enzymes in the food-enzyme stomach enough time to digest and liquefy the food mass sufficiently to allow it to flow down where the pepsin awaits the protein part of it. The data plainly show that the human stomach is really two stomachs with separate functions and that humans, in common with thousands of other species, have been provided with the means of letting outside enzymes help with the burdens of digesting food. The data further show that cathepsin in food, and other outside enzymes operating at the same pH range as gastric cathepsin are ready to step in and allow the enzyme potential to make fewer digestive enzymes and more metabolic enzymes as needed. In other parts of the book I have shown that starch is normally and efficiently digested in the stomach and that enzyme fractions in saliva, in food, or in supplements can be reactivated and recovered in the intestines. We must concede that it required more than a little scheming by evolution to contrive this wonderful coordination and achieve such perfect symbiosis. Unfortunately, human beings make little effort to get the benefit of such outside enzymes as are found in raw food and supplements.

Figure 4.2

DIAGRAMMATIC REPRESENTATIONS OF
FOOD-ENZYME STOMACHS

In animals and humans alike, food-enzyme stomachs are always the first stop stations of food in its journey through the digestive tract. In addition to those listed below, numerous species of rodents, monkeys, and bats have cheek pouches and hip pouches to keep food moist and warm so that its food enzymes can perform predigestion.

Food-Enzyme Stomachs Illustrated as Squares in the Following

HUMAN

In humans, the cardiac portion is the food-enzyme stomach.

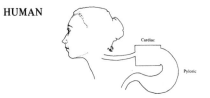

CHICKEN

In seed-eating birds such as the chicken and the pigeon, the crop is the food-enzyme stomach.

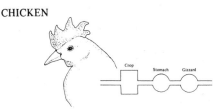

COW

In ruminative animals such as the cow and the sheep, there are three food-enzyme stomachs:

1st – Rumen
2nd – Reticulum
3rd – Omasum

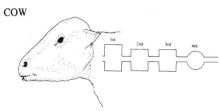

WHALE

In Cetacea such as the dolphin and whale, the 1st stomach is the food-enzyme stomach.

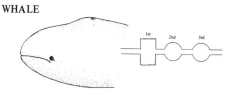

Gray's Anatomy cites the authority Walter B. Cannon who demonstrated that the human stomach "consists of two parts physiologically distinct." *Gray's Anatomy* states: "The cardiac portion of the stomach is a food reservoir in which salivary digestion continues; the pyloric portion is the seat of active gastric digestion. There are no peristaltic waves in the cardiac portion." Predigestion by exogenous (outside) enzymes is widespread in nature. Our enzyme potential has other and more useful and taxing work to do than merely making endogenous digestive enzymes to digest food.

COMPARATIVE ANATOMY AND PHYSIOLOGY

Before we move to the Law of Adaptive Secretion of Digestive Enzymes, I wish to present one more interesting piece of evidence showing the differences in gastrointestinal anatomy of various animals and man. Mankind's change in diet from mostly uncooked to cooked foods has probably resulted in changes in the structure of our gastrointestinal tract beyond the stomach; specifically, the appendix and cecum (the beginning of the large intestine) play an active role in digestion in many herbivorous animals but have atrophied in humans. Most vegetables eaten by man are first cooked and contain no enzymes. Could the appendix and cecum of humans be food-enzyme stomachs which have shrunk for lack of use?

For many years I have been gathering data in the periodical scientific literature on the weight and measurement of parts of the gastrointestinal tract in man and animals. Although the data are incomplete, they have been tabulated in Tables 4.2 and 4.3 in ascending and descending order. Such treatment has been devised to enable a better evaluation of the role that function plays in ordering structure.

Table 4.2

PROPORTION OF LENGTH OF SMALL AND LARGE INTESTINE TO TOTAL LENGTH OF INTESTINE

Species	Authority	Year
Seal	Owen	1866
Whale, Piked	Hunter	1840
Hippopotamus	Crisp	1867
Dolphin, Plot. gang.	Takahashi	1972
Dolphin	Anderson	1868
Rat, Norway, wild	E. Howell	1968
Rat, Norway, lab.	Richter et al.	1947
Great Ant Eater	Owen	1862
Hippopotamus	Chapman	1881
Lion	Hunter	1861
Whale, Fin	Murie	1865
Dog, hunting, zoo	Crisp	1855
Goose, domestic	Robertson et al.	1965
Monkey, insects & fruit	Fooden	1964
Cat, domestic	Latimer	1937
Cat, domestic	Latimer	1937

One of the objects of publishing these tables is to induce anatomists to participate in organ-weight research on man and animals and contribute their findings to the scientific literature. I am aware that it has been determined that the length of the intestine is shorter in living man than after death. Relaxation of the musculature after death causes the intestine to become longer. But this should not disturb the relative values in the tables because its influence is uniform.

Knowing the habits, manner of life, diet, and gastrointestinal anatomy of animal species enables professionals to structure the best diet for human beings to promote health and longevity. Table 4.2 has been compiled from isolated reports over many years and is presented to encourage anatomists and physiologists to perform more research which might add to our understanding of the significance of this data. In many cases only one specimen was reported in Table 4.2 and it was necessary to search literature more than 100 years old to find the report.

We can see in Table 4.3 yet another confirmation that food-enzyme stomachs are an integral part of the digestive system. In this table, the length of the cecum has been arranged in descending values in the entries, to indicate its possible role in gastrointestinal comparative physiology. Table 4.3 shows that the horse and rabbit are in the upper part of the descending "cecal scale," while sheep and cattle are lower

Body Weight Grams	Body Length mm.	No. of Specimens	Sex	Small Int. %	Large Int. %
—	914	1	—	95	5
—	—	1	—	91	9
339,750	1,727	1	—	91	9
—	1,185	3	—	90	10
—	2,381	1	—	89	11
269	223	3	M & F	89	11
200-249	—	58	M & F	88	12
28,123	1,397	1	F	88	12
249,480	1,676	1	F	86	14
—	—	1	—	86	14
408,420,000	18,288	1	M	86	14
—	—	1	—	85	15
4,900	—	5	M	85	15
675	267	above 10	M & F	85	15
2,821	—	52	M	84	16
2,445	—	52	F	84	16

Table **4.2,** *Continued*

Species	Authority	Year
Dog, domestic	E. Howell	1925
Wolf, zoo	Crisp	1855
Chicken, domestic	Kaupp	1918
Mouse, Albino, lab.	Loewe	1937
Man; Burma	Castor	1912
Man, Hindu	Castor	1912
Man, American Negro	Lamb	1893
Man, India	Deakin	1883
Swine, domestic	McMeekin	1940
Dog, hunting	Hunter	1861
Camel, zoo	Crisp	1865
Rat, Alexan., herbivore	Richter et. al.	1947
Man, German	Bryant	1924
Cow, Jersey, dairy	Swett et al.	1937
Cow, Holstein, dairy	Swett et al.	1937
Man, German	Dreike	1895
Swine, domestic	Sisson	—
Man, English	Underhill	1955
Ox, domestic	Sisson	—
Sheep, domestic	Wallace	1948
Monkey, frugivore	Fooden	1964
Snapping Turtle	Owen	1866
Monkey, leaf & fruit	Fooden	1964
Reptile, insectivore	Lonnberg	1902
Horse, domestic	Sisson	1910
Monkey, frugivore	Fooden	1964
Chimpanzee	Sonntag	1923
Rhinoceros	Owen	1862
Rhinoceros	Owen	1862
Reptile, herbivore	Lonnberg	1902
Rhinoceros	Garrod	1873
Rabbit, domestic	E. Howell	1934
Elephant	Crisp	1855
Guinea Pig, lab.	Eaten	1938
Guinea Pig, lab.	Eaten	1938
Drill	Sonntag	1922
Marsupial, Phal. vul.	Todd	1847
Gerbil, lab.	Kramer	1964
Gerbil, lab.	Kramer	1964
Gopher	Owen	1866
Marsupial, Koala	Todd	1847

Body Weight Grams	Body Length mm.	No. of Specimens		Sex	Small Int. %	Large Int. %
16,330	737		1	F	83	17
—	851		1		83	17
—	—		—	—	83	17
24	—		144	M	83	17
54,432	—		100	M	83	17
50,803	—		63	M	82	18
—	—		48	M & F	82	18
—	—		100	M & F	82	18
100,000	—		1	M	82	18
—	940		1	—	82	18
—	—		—	F	81	19
200-249	—		50	M & F	81	19
—	—		160	M & F	80	20
412,767	—	above	214	F	80	20
573,791	—	above	181	F	79	21
—	—		171	M & F	79	21
—	—		—	—	79	21
—	—		100	M & F	78	22
—	—		—	—	78	22
—	—		—	—	77	23
2,950	407	above	1	—	77	23
1,052	—		1	—	76	24
6,980	537	above	1	M & F	75	25
—	93		25	—	75	25
—	—		—	—	74	26
1,740	346	above	1	M & F	72	28
—	597		1	F	70	30
—	2,743		1	F	69	31
—	4,267		1	M	68	32
—	267		6	—	68	32
—	2,451		1	F	66	34
2,378	457		1	M	65	35
2,366,925	—		1	F	65	35
992	—		89	M	60	40
943	—		26	F	62	38
—	748		1	—	57	43
—	41		2	—	48	52
101	138	above	42	M	36	64
87	132	above	49	F	36	64
2,949	—		1	—	34	66
—	49		1	—	31	69

down. The horse and rabbit have small, single stomachs, while sheep and cattle have four stomachs, three of which depend on exogenous enzymes to digest food.

Table 4.3

PROPORTION OF LENGTH OF CECUM
TO TOTAL LENGTH OF INTESTINE

Species	Authority	Year
Gerbil, lab.	Kramer	1964
Gerbil, lab.	Kramer	1964
Marsupial, Koala	Todd	1847
Marsupial, Phal. vul.	Todd	1847
Rabbit	Dukes (Colin)	1947
Rabbit, lab.	E. Howell	1934
Goose, domestic	Roberson et al.	1965
Rhinoceros	Garrod	1873
Monkey, frugivore	Fooden	1964
Elephant	Crisp	1855
Monkey, frugivore	Fooden	1964
Horse	Sisson	1910
Monkey, leaf and fruit	Fooden	1964
Monkey, Spider	Flower	1872
Dog	Crisp	1855
Monkey, insects and fruit	Fooden	1964
Monkey, leaves	Ayer	1948
Drill	Sonntag	1922
Ox	Dukes (Colin)	1947
Dog	Sisson	1910
Baboon	Flower	1872
Sheep	Palsson et al.	1952
Chimpanzee	Sonntag	1923
Sheep	Palsson et al.	1952
Sheep	Wallace	1948
Ox	Sisson	1910
Dolphin	Anderson	1875
Swine	Sisson	1910
Swine	McMeekan	1940
Dolphin	Takahashi et al.	1972
Lion	Hunter	1861
Whale	Hunter	1840
Man	Cunningham	1914

The enormous ceca of the horse and rabbit digest large amounts of plant foods that their small stomachs cannot handle. This digestion in food-enzyme stomachs at the end of the small intestine must be done by the enzymes supplied by raw food because the cecum has no digestive enzymes of its own. Intestinal bacteria can also be expected to contribute enzyme action in the cecum. A biological law

Body Weight Grams	Body Length mm.	No. of Specimens	Sex	Small Int. %	Large Int. %	Cecum %
101	138	above 42	M	0.362	0.163	0.475
87	132	above 49	F	0.364	0.161	0.475
—	49	1	—	0.313	0.425	0.262
—	41	2	—	0.477	0.364	0.159
—	—	—	—	0.610	0.280	0.110
2,378	457	1	M	0.641	0.244	0.097
4,900	—	5	M	0.850	0.068	0.082
—	2,451	1	F	0.655	0.291	0.054
2,950	407	above 1	F	0.766	0.182	0.052
2,366,925	—	1	F	0.649	0.307	0.044
1,740	346	above 1	M & F	0.720	0.229	0.051
—	—	—	—	0.726	0.238	0.036
6,980	537	above 1	M & F	0.748	0.220	0.032
—	—	1	—	0.822	0.148	0.030
—	—	1	—	0.824	0.148	0.028
675	267	above 10	M & F	0.854	0.118	0.028
—	—	1	—	0.775	0.200	0.025
—	749	1	—	0.565	0.414	0.021
—	—	—	—	0.81	0.17	0.02
—	—	—	—	0.836	0.145	0.019
—	—	1	—	0.687	0.294	0.019
65,685	—	2	F	0.772	0.212	0.016
—	597	1	F	0.703	0.282	0.015
97,622	—	2	M	0.779	0.207	0.014
—	—	—	—	0.773	0.215	0.012
—	—	—	—	0.778	0.210	0.012
—	2,381	1	—	0.890	0.098	0.012
—	—	—	—	0.786	0.203	0.011
100,000	—	1	—	0.816	0.174	0.010
—	—	3	—	0.899	0.093	0.008
—	—	1	—	0.857	0.135	0.008
—	—	1	—	0.906	0.088	0.006
—	—	—	—	0.800	0.192	0.008

can be seen to operate; vegetable eaters with one stomach have enormous ceca; those with four stomachs have small ceca.

The gerbil and koala are other animals with large ceca. Gerbils are rodents native to Asia and Africa, which are used in laboratory research. The koala is the famous Australian "bear" almost exterminated for its fine fur. As Table 4.3 shows, these animals have such huge ceca they almost compare with their intestine in size. I am inclined at this time to include the ceca of the horse, rabbit, gerbil, and koala in the list of food-enzyme stomachs, subject to change in the light of future evidence. Although textbooks state that the functions of the cecum and its appendix are unknown, Table 4.3 indicates that the cecum is indeed a digestive organ. Most of the vegetables eaten by man are cooked and contain no enzymes to help their digestion. Perhaps that is the reason his cecum has atrophied and that man is so low in the "cecal scale."

PREDIGESTION AND THE LAW OF
ADAPTIVE SECRETION OF DIGESTIVE ENZYMES

During the course of this narrative I have made references a number of times to the Law of Adaptive Secretion of Digestive Enzymes. It is important to understand precisely what this means so that your knowledge of the intimate details of the enzyme family will not be spotty, nor of their private lives, faulty. At the beginning of this century there was widespread ignorance of the nature of enzymes. During this period of information poverty, Professor B.P. Babkin announced some preliminary data on enzymes which was published in the *Transactions of the Imperial Medical Academy*, Saint Petersburg, Russia, in 1904 and has become known as the Theory of the Parallel Secretion of Enzymes. This theory held that the three main digestive enzymes, amylase, protease, and lipase, were secreted at the same strength, even if only one of them were needed and called for by the food eaten.

What kind of physiological law and order would prompt all of the enzymes to be secreted at the same strength when only starchy food is eaten? One would expect that a baked potato would stimulate only the secretion of amylase, which is the enzyme needed for starch digestion. If meat were consumed, only protease would be secreted in quantity; with amylase and lipase in token amounts. And so on. But the Babkin theory held that all three enzymes were secreted in the same strong concentration even if only one of them were needed to digest food. This mistaken idea was the product of a basic ignorance of the nature and intrinsic value of enzymes to life, health, and disease control. Nevertheless, Professor Babkin issued a further report which was published in 1935 in the *Journal of the American Medical Association* in which he reiterated: "The concentration of only one (lipase) of the three principal enzymes of the pancreatic juice was determined, since these enzymes are secreted in parallel concentration by the pancreatic gland in the dog, in man, and in the rabbit." It cannot be explained why this theory gained such wide acceptance and had such a tenacious hold on science.

We can say that this acceptance of a false doctrine for so many years is a tragedy, an unpardonable oversight by science. I would say it set back acceptance of the philosophy of enzyme nutrition 50 years, for the Theory of Parallel Secretion encouraged the idea that enzymes are expendable, that the body can waste them with impunity, and that they are utterly unimportant. A more fictitious chain of contradictions is hard to imagine.

Now let us see what the scientific periodical literature has to say about how the body responds to requests for digestive enzymes. A perusal of the information collected over many years, which is presented in Table 4.4, will show that as early as 1907, the Law of Adaptive Secretion of Digestive Enzymes was already being confirmed. Some of the results may need a word of explanation: for example, the absence of amylase in the whale's pancreas can be expected because the whale eats no starch and has no need for amylase; and the hen eats starchy food, which explains why Hirata found 800 times more amylase in its pancreas than in that of the cat, which does not eat starch in nature.

Further confirmation of the theory of Adaptive Secretion came in 1930 (prior to Babkin's second report), when it was shown that the feces of meat-eating animals had much trypsin and little amylase, while the feces of carbohydrate eaters had much amylase and little trypsin. Because of the eminence of Professor Babkin, I feel it is necessary to go into considerable detail in presenting evidence bearing on enzyme secretion.

Professor Babkin's 1935 report in the *Journal of the American Medical Association* mentioned none of this evidence which doomed his theory of parallel secretion. It seems to me that he grossly undervalued enzymes and had not done his homework. I can quote at least twenty more authorities whose work supports the adaptive secretion law. If you take in outside enzyme reinforcements for predigestion, the Law of Adaptive Secretion of Digestive Enzymes and your food-enzyme stomach will become your best friends. They will enable you to allocate fewer of your personal enzymes for digestion and more of them for metabolism. This will keep your whole body operating to make you feel well, prevent disease, and help correct the malfunctions causing human ailments. Good enzyme nutrition needs outside enzyme reinforcements. Don't disappoint nature—give her the outside enzyme reinforcements your primordial ancestors had been getting for millions of years. Good enzyme nutrition is imperative, especially if you are a practitioner of the fatal process, which will be our next topic of discussion.

Table 4.4

**EVIDENCE SUPPORTING THE LAW OF
ADAPTIVE SECRETION OF DIGESTIVE ENZYMES**

Year	Authority	Conclusion
1907	L. G. Simon	Human saliva is more powerful in amylase on a carbohydrate (starch) diet than on a mixed diet. On a protein diet salivary amylase is weaker than on a carbohydrate diet.
1909	Neilson and Lewis	In human subjects a carbohydrate diet increases salivary amylase, while a protein diet decreases it.
1910	G. Hirata	The concentration of amylase in the pancreas of hens is 800 times more than in the cat.
1925	M. Takata	Amylase is absent in the pancreas of the whale.
1927	B. Goldstein	Content of lipase, trypsin, and amylase in human pancreatic juice depends on kind of food.
1930	Georgievskii and Andreev	In dogs with fistulae, the amylase content of intestinal juice is directly proportional to the amount of starch.
1930	Krzywanek and Bedi-iu Schakir	Feces of carnivores and omnivores contain much trypsin (which acts on protein) and little amylase, whereas those of herbivores contain little trypsin but much amylase.
1932	Andreev and Georgievskii	In dogs, the amylase content of intestinal juice depends on the carbohydrate content of the diet, being least on a meat diet and increasing with increase in carbohydrate.

Table 4.4, *Continued*

Year	Authority	Conclusion
1935	Bykov and Davydov	In a patient with a pancreatic fistula, a fat diet increases the lipase content of pancreatic juice, a carbohydrate diet the amylase content, and a meat diet the trypsin.
1935	Vasyutochkin and Drobintzeva	In human pancreatic juice obtained by fistulae, lipase increases with a fat diet, amylase on a carbohydrate diet, and trypsin on meat.
1935	L. Abranson	The enzyme content of the pancreatic secretion adjusted itself to the character of the diet, in a study of 28 human subjects.
1937	T. Muto	In a dog with a permanent pancreatic fistula, the pancreatic juice contains more trypsin after a protein-rich diet, and more amylase after a carbohydrate-rich diet.
1943	Grossman, Greengard, and Ivy	Using 162 white rats, it was found that on a high-carbohydrate diet there is a pronounced increase in amylase, and a decrease in trypsin. A high-protein diet results in greatly increased trypsin (These results were obtained by measuring the enzymes in the pancreatic tissue of the rats. The amount of enzymes in the tissue is paralleled by the amount found in the pancreatic juice.)
1947	J. Monad	The phenomenon of enzyme adaptation leads to a conservation of energy, and a decrease in the concentration of an enzyme may increase the amount of other enzymes more essential under the circumstances.
1954	D.K. Kuimov	In pancreatic juice of sheep, the concentration of lipolytic, proteolytic and amylolytic enzymes depends on the diet.
1964	Abdeljlil and Desnuelle	In both pancreatic tissue and pancreatic juice of rats on a starch-rich diet, amylase is two to three time higher than controls on a normal mixed diet.
1967	Roy, Campbell and Goldberg	In 17 ileostomy patients, raising the protein intake from 40 to 90 grams per day caused an increase in trypsin output by 69.5 percent and an increase in chymotrypsin output by 26 percent.

5

The Fatal Process

ENZYME-DEFICIENT DIETS, REFINED FOODS, AND ORGAN IMBALANCES

The last 100 years have seen a dramatic change in our food supply in America. The refining and otherwise processing of food, and "improved" cooking methods like microwave ovens and gas and electric ranges, have rendered the modern diet enzyme-deficient due to the effective destruction of the enzymes in foods by these appliances and processes. Unfortunately, little attention has been paid to how the lack of enzymes in our food relates to imbalances in our organs, and the resulting diseases. In this chapter I will present the history of cooking and show how and why the cooking and refining of foods is responsible for the development of various illnesses and health problems plaguing humans today.

ENZYME-DEFICIENT DIETS

Scientists believe that animal life goes back several hundred million years. Yet even the most primitive living form in the evolutionary scale took in enzymes as part of its food. It could be no other way, because enzymes are components of living matter. No living organism, either animal or vegetable, could exist without hundreds of enzymes in its make-up. Throughout all of the millions of years of evolutionary development, countless branches of the animal kingdom ate enzymes as an integral part of the diet. Considering this past history of several hundred millions of years, is it not more than a little unusual, more likely bordering on reckless and dangerous, for modern man to rather abruptly and almost completely remove the hundreds of food enzymes from his diet? We must learn to think of enzymes—food enzymes—as a part of our food. It may not be easy to prove all of the many functions food enzymes are suspected of performing for their host, but it is impossible to imagine or prove that when in the presence of a suitable substrate within the living organism, they do not act on it in the manner characteristic of endogenous enzymes.

In 1925, a pharmacist named Nels Quelvi appears to have become highly enthused and intrigued about enzymes, for he published a book entitled *Enzyme Intelligence, Illustrating That Enzymes and Ferments are the Ultimate, Indestructible and Invisible Units of Life and are Conscious and Intelligent.* Some of his concepts, which once appeared plausible, have not been supported by developments in science. At the time, however, I wrote to Mr. Quevli and bought copies of his pioneering work. Scientists now know that enzymes, far from being indestructible, are highly fragile things. They suffer from excessive light and pressure, but especially from heat. If we entertain any suspicion that food enzymes play a part in human physiology, we had better be aware of the fact that the heat employed in all manner of cooking, even the mildest kind, kills 100 percent of food enzymes. That leaves the vast majority of the human race with what I have termed the minus diet; i.e., food without enzymes

There are many people who are quite satisfied that when an element—any element—is found to be a normal ingredient in food, that element should be consumed and treasured as a necessary factor in the diet. These people believe that if any food element is left out of the diet it may trigger an unwholesome, or even a pathogenic, body reaction, and that this expectation will be confirmed when the tired machinery of scientific research finally completes an investigation. Other people, mainly scientists, ask for proof as to the exact function of each food element in the body of the host organism before accepting it as a necessary food element, but do not command anyone in possession of the necesary facilities to conduct a search for evidence. Before this proof is forthcoming they are not concerned whether or not the organism gets all of the natural elements bequeathed by food. *Enzyme Nutrition* was written to fill a distressing void which the substance of the book fully illustrates.

Food enzymes have always existed in all foods and for that reason are believed by many to fulfill a need in nutrition. The believers are thousands of people I have met during some 60 years who contend no one has the knowledge to say that taking something away from food is "safe," or adding a foreign element to food is "safe." Lifespan studies on short-lived creatures over extended periods are necessary to throw light on these matters. The believers ask for proof as to how such highly active materials as food enzymes could be prevented from acting upon their own food substrates when eaten as a part of normal food. Therefore the burden of proof is as much on one side as it is on the other. It is necessary to show that man could make the transition from a primitive consumer of raw food and its enzymes to a modern cooked, enzyme-free diet without becoming host to the swarm of diseases that plague modern man. It is decidedly unbecoming for those possessing the tools of science to close their eyes to the possibility that those diseases which are human trademarks, such as cancer and heart disease, are the products of disturbed metabolism induced partly by the hidden machinations of food enzyme deficiency.

THE DISCOVERY OF COOKING

Let the reader consider that a human baby, like an infant animal, is given raw food having a full complement of enzymes, from the breasts of its mother. If it needed cooked food for survival, it would have been provided with it. But in fact, a newborn infant has no need for cooked food. A cooking stove, which is a human invention, does not come permanently attached as a part of the anatomy of a newly born infant!

Perhaps early man first learned about fire in equatorial jungles by having to cope with forest fires caused by lightning. Or he may have gotten some original education by coming close to hot lava flows from an active volcano. Later, man's original dread of fire turned to awe and pleasant anticipation after he tasted the carcasses of burned and roasted animal victims of these occasional natural disasters. Early man had several million years to get acquainted with fire and the use of stone, bone, and wood implements. This knowledge enabled him to add larger animals to his food supply. While his teeth or nails were of no use in ripping off the hide to get at the meat, the sharpened edges of abundant stones served well. Gradually, a new world beckoned: concentrated protein from the meat; clothing and shelter from the skins. Man could now migrate to sparsely populated northern regions, where he used warm clothing and made fire when needed. Every invention must be suspected of harboring potential health hazards unless proven otherwise. It is the misuse of fire by man in the form of cooking that I have called the fatal process. We will see why.

Any kind of heat treatment of food in the kitchen destroys enzymes. Slow or fast baking, slow or fast boiling, stewing, and frying all destroy 100 percent of the enzymes in food. Vigorous boiling takes place at 212° F. Frying is done at a much higher temperature, and in addition to destroying enzymes, it also damages protein, or forms new chemical compounds with unknown and possibly pathogenic possibilities, imposing still more burden upon the metabolic enzymes. Although baking takes place at 300° to 400° F, it is in dry heat, so the effect is no more destructive than at boiling temperatures. Enzymes are completely destroyed at *all* of these temperatures, however.

When I was in active medical practice, I developed a special electrothermotherapy immersion apparatus to apply high temperature treatment to specific parts of the body to stimulate local enzyme activity. This activity increases two to three times for every 10° F increase in local temperature. I modified some of this apparatus to permit experiments to determine the thermal death point of protoplasm (living matter), and found that immersion in water at 118° F destroyed enzymes in a half-hour. The temperature of 118° F also blistered the skin, and prevented subsequent germination of seeds when they were immersed for a half-hour. Comparing 118° F with any of the cooking temperatures, you can see that the enzymes in foods have not the slightest chance of escaping destruction under any kind of kitchen heat exposure.

In 1937, Kohman, Eddy, White, and Sanborn, Columbia University, published a paper entitled "Comparative Experiments With Canned, Home Cooked and Raw Food Diets," *Journal of Nutrition* 14:9-19 (1937). It turned out that the canned food eaters were the heavyweights. Canned food, which must be cooked at high heat to preserve it, exerted a powerful stimulating effect on the endocrine chain, promoting a large body weight increase. (The endocrine chain is a system of glands that help to regulate body function.) I believe this is the proper way to interpret the results of this experiment, although I am aware that another interpretation is usually employed. To say that cooking improves utilization and absorption misses the point. Is anyone so naive as to insist that we can improve on a process that has kept a vast population of organisms living out their lives for millions of years without the aid of the cookstove? If utilization of raw foodstuffs proceeded at a normal rate for these millions of years and we step in and do something to food, such as cooking it, which increases its utilization and absorption beyond the normal, this amounts to a perversion. If obesity is the result, it certainly is not wholesome. And it does not require deep insight to perceive that the evil consequences of such an assault on the endocrine balance may later hand us a legacy of many apparently unrelated pathological entities.

The Enzyme Bank Account

In the animal kingdom enzyme reinforcements are coming in continuously through the food. But in man, the trillions of cells in the whole body are called upon to supply the entire enzyme requirements, since our enzyme intake is practically nil. This is because almost no uncooked food that is high in calories is used. Foods low in calories, such as raw salad, vegetables, and juicy fruits, are also low in enzyme content. We will discuss this matter in greater detail in Chapter 6, but for now let us discuss it briefly. Let us say that a certain diet has a value of 2,500 calories each day. If it included a lettuce salad, an apple, and an orange, that would break down into about 200 calories of raw food that supplies enzymes. The calories in the salad dressing must be counted amongst the cooked calories. The result: 2,300 cooked calories that have had all of their enzymes taken from them, and only 200 calories supplying some enzymes. But I doubt that very many people take in as many as 200 raw calories a day. Ready-made orange juice would count with cooked calories.

It should not be hard to see how the enzyme bank account of the body can get out of balance; heavy withdrawals, skimpy deposits. As I pointed out earlier, if people spend their enzymes rapidly, their life does not last as long as it would if they used enzymes more frugally. Like an indulgent parent who caters unstintingly to demanding offspring, the body responds generously to calls for digestive enzymes. The remarkable thing about the eventual bankruptcy of the enzyme account is that it can proceed quite painlessly, without immediate symptoms. Digestion of food takes a high priority and acts as a powerful stimulus in the demand for enzymes. If this function takes more than its rightful share, the other organs and tissues must try to get along with the remaining capacity. The only warning may be a belated malfunction or breakdown in some organ far removed from the digestive tract. But the diagnostician unaware of the importance of enzyme nutrition would have difficulty in connecting such a referred process to the true, underlying cause. This is how an assortment of human ailments may get started.

What does all this mean? Shortened lifespan, inferior health of the organs, and nagging illnesses; and all due to an enzyme-deficient diet. Let us now take a closer look at the evidence.

PHYSIOLOGICAL CHANGES ACCOMPANYING CIVILIZATION

Now, I will unearth a tomb of buried facts which may disturb or shock the reader. We have been conditioned to equate civilization with an increase in the size of the human brain. The skull of *Homo sapiens* is much more capacious than fossil skulls of our ancestors lower in the evolutionary scale. Writers in a former era used to hypothesize that the brain of future man would become so large, while his lower extremities dwindled from lack of use, that a special personal cart would be needed by each individual to carry the monstrous head about! It should prove more than a little disquieting, then, when we learn that these authors were wrong. Fossil skulls have been found of the Neanderthal (cave) man only 50,000 to 100,000 years old, in which you could put the human brain and have room to spare. This means that some cavemen had bigger brains than ours, although it is likely that our brains are larger in the frontal lobes (the seat of the intellectual faculties). Does civilization make a smaller brain? You will have to form your own conclusion on this matter after I present some pertinent evidence.

As we will see, there are some indications that life in the wild provides certain kinds of cerebral gymnastics missing from the protected arena of civilized life. Charles Darwin noted that the domesticated rabbit has a smaller brain than his wild cousin. Donaldson, one of the first scientists to work with the white rat in the laboratory, wrote that the brain weight or cranial capacity of the rat, guinea pig, lion, rabbit, and fox is less in the captive than in the corresponding wild creature, the deficiency in domesticated guinea pigs being about 7 percent. The size of the brain of the wild Norway rat exceeds that of the laboratory white rat by 7–15 percent when animals of corresponding body weight are compared.

The accompanying table (Table 5.1) is abridged from my more detailed organ weight tables. The brain weight is given as a percentage of the body weight. It is seen that the brains of wild meadow mice are twice as heavy as those of tame laboratory mice. In the comparison with domestic animals, I have chosen somewhat similar wild species with similar body weight. If organ weight data are to have any validity, only animals of corresponding body weight can be compared. In each of these comparisons of the domestic sheep, cattle, and horse with its wild counterpart, it can be seen that the brain of the wild creature is heavier. Each of the figures is an average or mean of many specimens.

Table 5.1

BRAIN WEIGHTS OF WILD AND DOMESTICATED ANIMALS

	Authority	Body Weight Grams	Sex	Brain (% of Body Weight)
Mouse, wild, Canada	Crile and Quiring	23.7	M	2.78
Mouse, wild, Canada	Crile and Quiring	22.9	F	2.82
Mouse, wild, Ohio	Crile and Quiring	27.9	M	2.65
Mouse, wild, Ohio	Crile and Quiring	25.2	F	2.85
Average, 204 wild mice		*24.9*		*2.78*
Mouse, laboratory	Marshal et al.	35.0	—	1.34
Mouse, laboratory	Anton	36.9	M	1.21
Mouse, laboratory	Anton	30.4	F	1.60
Average, 23 laboratory mice		*34.4*		*1.38*
Domestic Sheep	Howell	43,495	—	0.25
Wild Impala and Gazelle	Crile and Quiring	44,980	—	0.31
Domestic Cattle	Howell	486,611	—	0.08
Wild Buffalo and Wildebeest	Crile and Quiring	515,003	—	0.11
Domestic Work Horse	Crile and Quiring	270,500	—	0.17
Wild Zebra	Crile and Quiring	281,066	—	0.20

The first thought to pop into the mind as an explanation of the decrease in brain weight under domestication is that domestication breeds a more relaxed state of the nervous system. If the muscles stay relaxed and little used for a period they get smaller—they atrophy. Can we expect the brain to get larger, or even maintain its weight, when the nervous system is overwhelmed by the tranquilizing influence of civilization? In the wild state, animals are kept under pressure with the daily problems of finding food and shelter and confrontations with superior enemies. The brain must be kept in a state of keen efficiency in order to solve these problems. Benjamin Franklin has been credited with calling man a "tool-making animal." But was it not the tool that made modern man, causing the brain to enlarge, and transforming near man to early man? When the hand of "near man" began experimenting with sharp stones and clubs, cells in the brain developed more and more protoplasmic extensions and hence connections with other nerve cells in response to this new activity. Through a somewhat similar mechanism, the brains of idle laboratory mice increase in weight 2 to 3 percent when they are given interesting but perplexing tasks to perform and puzzles to solve.

The information and tables presented in this section on the comparative weight of the brain in various species and different environments will provide interested readers with a basis to evaluate facts and make judgments. While I leave definite conclusions to the reader, it appears to be true that domestication exerts a tranquilizing influence on mental activity in some ways, and thereby reduces brain size, perhaps only in certain parts of the brain. This evidence makes it quite clear that another factor must be considered as having a similar effect. When civilization took man and his domesticated animals under its umbrella, the food of all of these creatures became markedly changed. It no longer contained all of the elements it supplied for millions of years. The most profound deficiency was induced by use of fire. Students of this subject must take this factor into account in coming to any conclusions about brain size.

Nutrition and Brain Weight

Domestication introduces another factor which must not be overlooked—nutrition. The food of laboratory and domestic animals such as rats, mice, guinea pigs, hamsters, dogs, rabbits, monkeys, and cats, is a skeletonized factory product, either canned, granulated, or particled. No raw food is used in the standard diet; it is completely free of food enzymes. But it is armed to the hilt with various vitamins and minerals. Farm animals such as sheep, cattle, and horses also suffer some loss of food enzymes. Part of their diet is being increasingly supplied in the form of commercially processed food that has been heat-treated in the factory and lost its enzymes.

When rats are given a "factory" diet, body weight goes up and brain weight goes down. I have reached this conclusion by assessing more than 50 reports submitted in the scientific periodical literature over a number of years. The tables that follow present this information in succinct form.

The diet fed to laboratory rats has changed considerably. In the first quarter of this century, the rats were commonly fed a mixture of cooked and uncooked foods. Often table scraps were used. In some cases, a large amount of raw grain, either whole or ground, was included. The entries showed that at any age or level of body weight, from 54 to 340 grams, the brain weights on the factory diets were consistently lower.

This is illustrated in Tables 5.2 and 5.3. The first table shows that Sofia's rats in the year 1969 reached 270 grams in about one-quarter of the time required by Donaldson's Albinos of 1924, and in an even shorter period than that required by the Wild Norways. In a 1969 letter, Dr. Sofia stated that the diet of his rats was a commercial dry laboratory chow. At a body weight of 270 grams, the brains of Sofia's modern rats were 10 percent lighter than the Albinos of 1924 and almost 25 percent less in weight than Wild Norways. In Table 5.3, Sofia's 1969 rats had reached the maximum mature weight for body and brain at the age of 140 days, while the body and brain of the 1924 Albinos and Norways continued to grow for a period at least 4 times as long as Sofia's 1969 rats.

Table 5.2

INFLUENCE UPON RATE OF BODY GROWTH AND
BRAIN WEIGHT IN RATS RAISED UPON DIFFERENT DIETS

Strain	Authority	Year	Body Weight Grams	Brain Weight Grams	Age Days
Long Evans	Sofia	1969	270.0	1.730	70
Albino	Donaldson	1924	270.7	1.945	270
Wild Norway	Donaldson	1924	270.4	2.256	318

Table 5.3

BODY AND BRAIN WEIGHT IN RATS AT AGE 140 DAYS

Strain	Authority	Year	Body Weight Grams	Brain Weight Grams	Age Days
Long Evans	Sofia	1969	421	1.94	140
Albino	Donaldson	1924	211	1.88	140
Wild Norway	Donaldson	1924	165	2.07	140

In laboratory mice, brain weight can be changed in as little as one month. Drs. N.B. Marshall, S.B. Andrus, and J. Mayer of Harvard Medical School discovered how to make mice fat rapidly. As Tables 5.4-5.6 show, there were four groups of mice. The first group inherited a tendency toward fatness. They were subjected to autopsy at 12 to 16 weeks of age. The second group was sacrificed at the adult stage. The third group was made fat by injecting thioglucose which made a lesion in a particular area in the brain. In mice of the fourth group, surgical means were employed to implant a lesion in the same brain area.

In mice with surgically or chemically induced brain lesions, as in the Marshall et al. study, the liver heart, kidneys, and pancreas become enlarged. In a piece of research work done by a team long before the Marshall work, continuous intravenous injection of large amounts of dextrose (glucose) into 20 dogs caused death in all of them in 1 to 7

Table 5.4

BRAIN WEIGHTS IN NORMAL AND
CONGENITALLY OBESE YOUNG MICE

	Body Weight Grams	Brain Weight Grams	Brain Weight as %
Normal Mice	23.3	.377	1.6
Congenitally Obese Mice	46.9	.320	.7

At the same age, the congentially obese mice became twice as heavy in body weight as normal mice, while their brains were smaller than normal.

Table 5.5

BRAIN WEIGHTS IN NORMAL AND
CONGENITALLY OBESE ADULT MICE

	Body Weight Grams	Brain Weight Grams	Brain Weight as %
Normal Adult Mice	29.2	.409	1.4
Congenitally Obese Adult Mice	66.6	.343	.5

In adult mice, the gulf between the normal and congenitally obese in body weight and brain weight becomes wider.

Table 5.6

BRAIN WEIGHTS IN NORMAL ADULT MICE AND MICE WITH CHEMICALLY AND SURGICALLY INDUCED BRAIN LESIONS

	Body Weight Grams	Brain Weight Grams	Brain Weight as %
Normal Adult Mice	34.9	.469	1.3
Adult Mice with Chemical Lesion	55.9	.453	.8
Adult Mice with Surgical Lesion	54.9	.443	.8

In mice with chemically or surgically induced brain lesions, the body weights exceed the norm, but the brain weights decline.

REFERENCE: Marshall, N.B.; Andrus, S.B.; Mayer, J. *American Journal of Physiology* 189:343-346 (1957).

days. It also caused severe hemorrhage and destruction in the pituitary gland and pancreas, and marked liver enlargement. This and other experiments create a compelling reason to believe that the habitual use of refined sugars and other carbohydrates over long periods can create brain lesions similar to the brain lesions produced in the laboratory.

It is widely believed that obesity is a disease of civilization and is associated with adverse nutrition in which enzyme undernutrition is implicated. Thus it can be said that the brain becomes smaller both under the influence of civilization and obesity. The evidence creates strong suspicion that as a person puts on useless fat his brain gets smaller. It is a glorious thought that if you are overweight and take off 20 to 30 pounds through a diet containing 75 percent raw calories, you may add good weight to your brain for more brain power, and be in a better mental condition to deal with taxing business and personal problems.

Organ weight studies have shown over and over again that poor nutrition profoundly disturbs the weight of most of the endocrine glands (such as the pituitary, thyroid, and pancreas), as well as many organs. Obesity is accompanied by profound changes in endocrine and organ weights. Obesity *per se* is only the visible aspect of hidden, and far more serious pathological conditions. In Dr. Marshall's mice, the liver became greatly enlarged, while the heart, kidneys, and pancreas also became enlarged. There is strong evidence recorded in the periodical literature that heavy use of refined sugar causes pituitary lesions and perhaps brain lesions like those produced artificially by Marshall et al.

The damaging side effects of enzyme undernutrition are brought home when we start looking under the skin. You cannot see the damage on the outside; look inside. Consider the enlarged pancreas. A big thyroid is a goiter. That not only looks ugly, but is bad. An enlarged kidney, liver, or spleen is also bad. What about an enlarged heart? It can kill. An enlarged pancreas is also nothing to brag about because it is able to give away and waste more precious enzymes than a smaller one. Consequently, I do not want anyone to conclude that making fat rats with smaller brains is the sum total of damage the enzymeless diet does to a living organism.

It should be realized that a highly processed factory diet is not being used only on laboratory animals to sustain them during the course of various research. Exactly the same technology is applied to the production of pet foods coming from factories. And the "rat diet" was first used on people many years ago in the form of dry, highly refined processed breakfast cereals that still occupy huge spaces on the shelves of stores. An enzymeless diet must be suspected as a criminal element in any human ailment unless proven innocent by scientific research. It should be understood that the factory diet fed universally to laboratory animals and to pet dogs and cats is used, not because it measures up to the strict dictates of science, but as a matter of convenience.

To find out if any harm comes to us when we adopt the ways of civilization, we like to observe what happens to captive wild animals or domesticated animals. These creatures have to give up the customs and food of nature and eat what we choose to give them. We have seen that when animals are taken under our wing, they gain body weight and their brains lose weight. Now let us examine how the pancreas is affected by enzyme undernutrition.

Diet and Pancreas Size

Is the human pancreas too big? My organ weight tables say yes. The following is proof why. When there are no food enzymes in the food you eat to predigest it, your pancreas must enlarge to give out more internal enzymes to do the job. The pancreas itself is hale and hearty, but your organs and tissues must try getting along with fewer metabolic enzymes. This is precisely the situation that intractable ailments such as cancer, hypertension, heart disease, and arthritis need to get going. It is the machination of enzyme undernutrition at its worst. Everything in your body is continually wearing out and must be replaced. This is called metabolism and is a part of life. Metabolic enzymes do the work. You need plenty of them. You can conserve these good housekeepers by letting outside enzymes do what nature and millions of years of evolution have fitted them to do—predigest food.

The Pancreas and Enzyme Activity

The pancreas must send messages to all parts of the body looking for enzymes it can reprocess into digestive enzymes. It may even invade the warehouse of the precursors. In a pinch it will beg, borrow, or steal them. When it finds them it has work to do. Changing metabolic enzymes into digestive enzymes means extra work for the pancreas. It must get bigger, just as a muscle grows from more exercise. This enlargement may not harm the pancreas, but when it confiscates metabolic enzymes it punishes the whole body by depriving it of the mechanics every organ and cell needs to carry on their processes and functions. As far as your health is concerned, it makes no difference whether the pancreas surreptitiously remodels metabolic enzymes into digestive enzymes, or whether it confiscates the precursors of metabolic enzymes. Either way, your brain, heart, arteries, and all organs and tissues suffer from an enzyme labor shortage.

In Table 5.7 I call attention to some research by R.A. Dieterich et al. of an Alaskan college, in which the scientists captured wild mice before doing the dissection and determined the organ weights. They weighed many organs, but I reproduce only the weight of the pancreas, which is expressed as a percentage of the body weight in grams.

Table 5.7

**PANCREAS WEIGHT OF WILD MICE
COMPARED TO LABORATORY WHITE MICE**

Species	Authority	Body Weight Grams	Pancreas Weight %	Number of Specimens
8 Wild Species	Dieterich et al.	37.1	0.32	141
Laboratory Mice		30.8	0.84	11

In Table 5.7, the weight of the pancreas of laboratory mice is represented by the percentage 0.84, compared to 0.32 for the wild rodents. The laboratory mouse has a pancreas more than twice the weight of its wild counterpart. These figures tell the calamitous state of affairs existing in the body of the laboratory white mouse when it is made to exist on an enzymeless diet. When the pancreas of the laboratory mouse must get 2½ times larger than that of its wild cousins in order to badger enough enzyme precursors from the rest of the body to digest the food which should have been digested by food enzymes, you can see the magnitude and seriousness of this kind of painless mischief. I am using the mouse as an example, but the enzymelesss diet is supplied to all laboratory animals, and vigorously advertised for cats, dogs, and human beings. I really believe that this data is relevant to you, the reader. It is up to you to spread this word around so people will wake up to the underlying cause of our health problems.

Enzymeless Diet Produces an Enlarged Pancreas

Scientists always want overwhelming proof before accepting a new idea. So I shall present the Food Enzyme Concept from yet another angle. In the foregoing table I have compared the size of the pancreas in mice and shown that wild mice, eating raw food with its enzymes intact, use up much less of their enzyme power than laboratory mice whose factory food has no enzymes to help them go easy on their own enzyme power. I claim that this is the main reason wild animals have none of our diseases. To investigate this, the reader could make a nutritional experiment, feeding one group of mice a raw diet, and another group the same food cooked (and therefore enzymeless). A reasonable period to complete the job would be two months. The animals would then be dissected and each pancreas weighed. But all you have to do is read about this laborious experiment; the work has already been done.

In organ weight research, some scientists who wish to determine how large the organs are for various reasons include the pancreas, which is a gland, in the study. Unfortunately, many such scientific reports leave out the pancreas. In Table 5.8, I have taken figures on the weight of the pancreas of laboratory rats from Dr. H.H. Donaldson's book, *The Rat*, and data donated by a German scientist named Brieger, to a journal named *Wilhelm Roux Archiv für Entwicklungemechanik der Organism*. Brieger knew nothing of food enzymes but wanted to find out if there was a difference in the weight of the pancreas, liver, kidneys, and heart on a raw meat diet, a raw vegetable diet, and a raw mixed diet.

Table 5.8

ORGAN WEIGHT OF RATS ON RAW OR COOKED DIET
ONE GRAM PER 100 GRAMS OF BODY WEIGHT

Authority and Diet	Year	Body Weight Grams	Pancreas %	Liver %	Kidneys %	Heart %
H. Brieger, raw meat diet	1937	124.4	0.175	6.51	1.10	0.456
H. Brieger, raw vegetable	1937	125.0	0.159	5.82	0.738	0.403
H. Brieger, raw mixed diet	1937	126.0	0.161	6.45	0.984	0.406
H. Brieger, average of above	1937	125.1	0.165	6.26	0.941	0.422
H.H. Donaldson, random diet	1924	125.4	0.521	5.68	0.913	0.447

To reinforce Dr. Donaldson's figure on the percentage weight of the pancreas (it is also called relative weight) in laboratory rats, I present in Table 5.9 listings on the weight of the pancreas in laboratory rats. Each of these represents a piece of research work done by scientists for various reasons, and at different periods. Note the number

Table 5.9

ABSOLUTE AND RELATIVE WEIGHT OF PANCREAS OF RATS
ON LABORATORY DIET

Authority	Body Weight Grams	Number of Specimens	Sex	Pancreas Weight Grams	Pancreas Weight (% of Body Weight)
Hatai	223	6	M	1.10	0.494
Hatai	230	6	F	1.12	0.488
Hess and Root	248	16	M & F	0.874	0.352
Hess and Root	273	16	M & F	0.945	0.346
Hammett	258	121	M	0.820	0.317
Hammett	179	121	F	0.682	0.381
Jackson	389	6	M	1.05	0.270
Schingoethe et al.	468	8	M	—	0.395
Schingoethe et al.	300	8	F	—	0.519
Snook	615	4	M	3.25	0.528
Average of above	318			1.23	0.409
Donaldson's table	317		M & F	1.485	0.469
Brieger's average	125	58		0.207	0.165
Donaldson's table	125		M & F	0.714	0.521

of animals used for each research project. Brieger used 58. The weight
of other organs was reported but they were excluded from this table.

In comparing Brieger's figure of 0.165 with Donaldson's 0.521, it is
seen that the pancreas of the laboratory rat on a diet characterized by
enzyme undernutrition is more than 3 times larger than the pancreas
of laboratory rats eating food with all of its enzymes. In other words,
the pancreas of rats eating the poor diet wastes more than 3 times as
many enzymes as the pancreas of rats on the raw diet. The inferior
health of laboratory rats is not generally noticed because most of them
are used for only short periods to investigate matters not requiring
extended research, and then destroyed. But there have been some
rat colonies that were allowed to live until all of the rats died at the
end of their lifespans. When these rats were dissected, an astonishing
array of typically human degenerative diseases was revealed.

We can summarize from the preceding data that the present enzyme-deficient diet may be responsible for the reduction in brain
weight and size, unfavorable enlargement of the pancreas, wasting
of the precursors of metabolic enzymes, and many degenerative
trends. Added to the modern catastrophe called the stove are hundreds of food factories whose job it is to "refine" or denature foods.
In almost every case, refining eliminates much of the enzymes in
foods, and in many cases also adds potential carcinogens to them.
As a primary example of the refining farce, let's take a look at the
perversion of sugar cane and its disastrous effects on the body.

REFINED WHITE SUGAR—AN ARCH ENEMY

Table sugar (sucrose) has been condemned by dentists, nutritionists,
and physicians for scores of years. It is the greatest scourge that has
ever been visited on man in the name of food. Endocrinologists agree
that the endocrine system of glands and the nervous system cooperate
to regulate the appetite so that the right amount of the right kind of
food is taken in. Sugar spoils this fine balance. Being almost 100
percent "pure," this high-calorie dynamite bombs the pancreas and
pituitary gland into gushing forth a hyper-secretion of hormones comparable in intensity to that artificially produced in laboratory animals
with drugs and hormones. Sugar is the culprit the endocrinologists
have been looking for that has been throwing the finely regulated
endocrine balance completely out of kilter. In this context, E.A.H.Sims
and E.S. Horton, University of Vermont, wrote in a 1968 article in
the *American Journal of Clinical Nutrition*, "Endocrine and Metabolic

Adaptation to Obesity and Starvation," as follows: "Such mechanisms, if exaggerated or distored, could interfere with normal caloric balance." These are mild words for what sugar does after it is swallowed.

As Drs. Sims and Horton point out, with normal food that carries all needed nutritional factors, the glands know just when the body has had enough and will shut off the appetite just as abruptly as one would shut off a water faucet. But when sugar gets into the mouth and begins its evil machinations, it throws the endocrine switchboard into helter-skelter. The glands know the organism has been loaded up with a lot of calories but in spite of searchng, the nutrients that normally go along with the calories cannot be found in the body. So an order to take in more food, in the expectation of getting the important vitamins, minerals, and enzymes, is issued in the form of increased appetite. Don't let it fool you, the increased appetite sugar induces is not a call for more sugar or the foods that it contaminates, but for the missing nutrient factors that your body craves. Eating added sugar in various foods and drinks every day is a way of perpetuating chronic overstimulation of the pituitary and pancreas glands. The thyroid and adrenals also feel the brunt of the affront. The false craving and feeling of well-being sugar induces is on a par with the ecstasy experienced when dope takes command in a victim's body. Therefore, far overshadowing the damage resulting from sugar as a carrier of empty calories, is its capacity to destroy the delicate endocrine balance and inaugurate a train of pernicious consequences.

"Sugarization" is an inexpensive device to make many products acceptable to the palate. Everyone has heard of the "sugar-coated pill." That could mean a real medicinal tablet, or it could refer to a controversial proposition that is hard to swallow. A large segment of industry depends on sugar to help sell its products. Can you imagine gum without sugar? Or cola drinks? Unsugared cookies and cakes would remain unsold on the market shelves. Even inferior or unripe fruit can be doctored up with the white stuff to sell it.

Sugared cereal products and hundreds of other items are made by sugarization, accounting for an average consumption of 100 pounds each year for every man, woman, and child in the USA. If the government outlawed sugar, it would shake the foundations of American business. It remains to be seen whether the ultimate damage to twenty-first century man will accrue more from today's sugar eating or from the consumption of artificial sweeteners such as saccharine.

Four scientists, headed by Dr. J. Yudkin at the University of London, finished a check-up in 1968 on the reason why we have been swamped by certain types of heart disease for upwards of 30 years. Some doctors, including Yudkin, blamed exchanging a big share of carbohydrate in the diet for common table sugar and the products it adulterates, as a factor in many diseases. The London researchers persuaded 10 young male students to go on diets for 2 weeks. Fifty percent of the calories came from carbohydrates. In 5 subjects, all of the carbohydrate was common white sugar. In the other subjects, the carbohydrate was flour made into pancakes with no sugar at all. The other nutrients in the diet for the 10 subjects were meat, green vegetables, and fat. To make it interesting, all of the subjects were rewarded by allowing 9 percent of the total calories in the form of alcoholic drinks. At the end of one week the group using the sugar switched to the pancake diet, while the pancake group took sugar during meals, in beverages and in between meals. The amount of sugar was 1800 calories a day, no greater than many people normally consume.

Both diets raised cholesterol levels about 40 percent. There were some other changes in the blood chemistry. But the most startling finding was that in all 10 subjects sucrose appeared in the urine when they ate sugar. This finding means that sucrose had to be absorbed first into the blood. This experiment led the doctors to hint that possibly table sugar (sucrose) gets into the urine of millions of people. (Sucrose is not the same kind of sugar as that found in urine of diabetics. That sugar is known as dextrose or glucose.) The remarkable thing is that the textbooks teach that the intestinal membranes are so well policed that sucrose cannot sneak into the blood but must first be digested into dextrose. When sucrose gets in, it is pumped from head to toes over and over again in a few minutes. What it does to the organs and tissues is anybody's guess and these London doctors are more than a little concerned.

Sugar and Obesity

Two doctors who investigated why their stout patients did not know when to stop eating published their findings in 1970 under the heading, "Obesity; Absence of Satiety Aversion to Sucrose." Drs. M. Cabanac and R. Duclaux of the Laboratory of Physiology, Faculty of Medicine, Lyon, France, gave sugar taste tests to obese patients and persons of normal weight. There were 10 women averaging 184 pounds and 5 men averaging 205 pounds. There were also 6 women and 4 men of normal weight. The tests, which were rather involved, consisted essentially of having the subjects taste sucrose solutions of varying strength before and after swallowing a glass of dextrose after fasting for 12 hours. Before swallowing the dextrose, the taste of sucrose was pleasant to all 10 normal subjects, but after taking the dextrose the taste of the table sugar (sucrose) solution was disagreeable to all of them if it was made strong enough. On the contrary, the stout people did not seem to notice any unpleasantness, regardless of the degree of the sweet taste. The doctors concluded that in obese people, the internal signals regulating the intake of food have been deranged. Through medical sleuthing, the machinations of the seductive white granules in perverting the machinery of the body are being gradually uncovered.

While white table sugar has been looked down on, dextrose occupies a sort of ill-defined sanctified place in the dietary thinking of many people. Dextrose and glucose are two names for essentially the same thing, a castrated carbohydrate shorn of everything worthwhile constituting a food. The skeletonized ghost known as dextrose is no better a food than sucrose, since it too is refined. All food-like qualities, such as protein, fat, minerals, vitamins, and enzymes are removed during its processing from corn. Dextrose is cheap enough in price to sweeten anything an ambitious food processor might wish to foist upon the consumer. As we shall see in Chapter 6, dextrose can have detrimental effects. The food processing industry has no qualms about this, but the hitch to the wider use of dextrose is that it is only about half as sweet as sucrose.

Dextrose, which is made by boiling corn starch with acid, should be reserved for occasional use as temporary intravenous medicine in hospitals. The indictment against both table sugar and dextrose is strong enough to demand that both be placed off-limits to people. Let them be available only by prescription issued by a doctor. The chemists in the large food processing plants are very efficient people. They know their subjects from A to Z. But the last thing they can afford to be concerned about is the consumer's health. Oh yes, they will protect the public health from immediate poisoning and the like. But they do not worry about what goes on in a consumer's body after 20 years of eating their products. If the result is a killing disease, it is given a name on a death certificate as an established disease entity and no one suspects that food had anything to do with it.

Some Perils of Sugar Consumption

Bearing on the matter about the efficiency of food technologists in promoting their products is a report from England in the 1969 issue of *Nature*, a journal carrying a variety of scientific information from around the world. Two English chemists, M. Brook and P. Noel (1969) while evidently promoting a product, developed some information which should be passed on to candy and cake eaters. They went to the trouble of feeding 5 baboons for 26 weeks on 2 kinds of diets. One diet had sucrose as the carbohydrate ingredient and the other featured dextrose. At the end of the experimental period the abdominal fat was examined, and it was found that the sucrose produced 3 times as much fat as did dextrose—it was 3 times as fattening. The experimenters suggested that food processors take note of this matter and use dextrose in place of sucrose in supermarket foods. But from the standpoint of long-range human health, I have to conclude that such a substitution is on a par with exchanging a rattlesnake for a cobra as a bed partner.

At the Netherlands Institute of Nutriton, Department of Medicine, Amsterdam, Drs. L.M. Dalderup and W. Visser (1969) decided to find out about the effect of sugar on the length of life. To test it out they assembled two groups of albino rats equally divided between male and female; in all, there were 88 animals. Both groups were fed a human type heat-treated diet with addition of a small amount of fresh vegetables and bananas. In one group, however, table sugar (sucrose) was used to replace an equal amount of calories in the form of potato bread. The rats, who were three weeks old at the start of the experiment, lived on the diet for 364 days and then started to die off. All had died after 819 days. Those receiving sugar had their lives shortened by about 15 percent for males and 5 percent for females. All animals developed severe kidney disease, but the males receiving the sugar acquired the disease sooner. It is well known that kidney disease is common in rats on a heat-treated, enzyme-free diet that is standard for laboratory rats.

In *Guy's Hospital Reports* (1969) Dr. I. MacDonald, a physiologist at Guy's Hospital Medical School, analyzed the medical indictments against sugar in his report, "Sucrose—What Else Besides Caries?" In the 1971 issue of *Diabetologia*, Drs. A.M. Cohen and E. Rosenmann of the Hebrew University, Israel, reported feeding 8 rats on diets containing 79 percent dextrose and 10 rats on diets with 79 percent starch. On the sugar diets, the blood showed an impaired dextrose tolerance curve. People with diabetes will know what that means; i.e., a tendency to disturb the normal blood sugar level. In addition, 5 of the rats on the sugar diet developed bad kidney disease.

"Sweet Mystery of Life" was an editorial in the prestigious journal *Food and Cosmetics Toxicology* in 1971 which cited many columns in medical journals as implicating sugar as a causative factor in:

atherosclerosis, coronary (heart) disease, kidney disease, liver disease, shortening of lifespan, making blood platelets stick together, causing rise in serum triglycerides, and increasing desire for coffee and tobacco.

Food and Cosmetic Toxicology went on to suggest that the evidence is not complete enough to capture the backing of a majority of scientists. Here, as in a law court, the defendant is presumed innocent until proven guilty by established scientific procedures which move immoderately slow. You may have seen someone shot and killed by a defendant. But a conviction may be years away, or a technicality may result in outright freedom for the guilty party. As a parallel, it could require a hundred years to outlaw the oral ingestion of sugar. In the meantime, its evil machinations will continue to wreck the fabric of millions of bodies, which is especially distressing for the innocent young. As a small boy I ignorantly ate loads of sugar in the form of candy and pastries, much to my subsequent sorrow.

Sugar and Coronary Disease

In an article in the *American Heart Journal* (1970), Dr. J. Yudkin, University of London, stressed that facts continue to accumulate which do not support the concept that dietary fat is the major factor in coronary heart disease (disease of the coronary arteries, which supply blood directly to the heart). He explained that there has been a rise in sugar consumption in England and the USA some twenty times in the last two centuries. As in other countries, the rise in sugar consumption parallels the increase in coronary heart disease. Dr. T.L. Cleave in the *Lancet* (1968) compared the high incidence of diabetes and coronary disease in the Indians living in Natal (a province of South Africa), who consume 110 pounds of sugar each per year, to the low incidence of these diseases in Indians living in India and consuming only 12 pounds of sugar per year. Incidentally, the Natal Indians consume their fats mostly in the unsaturated form. Purified corn oil is a skeletonized unsaturated fat. Butter produced from certified raw milk is a natural saturated fat. From the standpoint of ultimate nutrition there is no choice between sugar and dietary fats. Both sugar and fats are skeletonized, that is, highly refined and providing only empty calories. Neither does any good. The only question can be which does the most harm. It is like a choice between the moon and Mars as a place to spend a delightful vacation, providing no respite from the prospect of danger and death.

The latest explosive evidence incriminating table sugar as the chief architect of heart disease comes from the University of Hawaii (1972). C.C. Brooks and his associates fed pigs high-sugar diets. Sixty-eight out of eighty pigs developed heart diesease in the left half of the heart. This backs up the contention of Dr. Yudkin and others have been making for many years. A remarkable added finding was that in pigs in which 10 percent of the sugar was replaced by coconut oil or beef tallow, the heart remained free from the endocarditis that afflicted the animals. This may confound those who have been apprehensive about fat in the diet.

In a report entitled, "How Sweet It Is!" Dr. R. Arky of Harvard Medical School (1972) pointed out that in the pre-insulin era, diabetes was regarded as a defect in carbohydrate metabolism, whereas now it has come to be recognized that it involves not only carbohydrate metabolism, but fat and protein also. Arky emphasized that it is important to maintain a normal body weight, and to change the type of carbohydrate from soft drinks, candies, and pastries, to a more wholesome variety.

THE DANGERS OF FOOD RADIATION

A fairly recent technological development that is highly touted by the Army, and is now being considered for widespread application to fresh produce, meats, and all otherwise uncooked foods sold in supermarkets, is radiation. The radiation preserves foods with dangerous rays (up to 4.5 rads of gamma radiation—10,000 times the dosage lethal to humans) and results in the wholesale destruction of all the enzymes and vital properties contained in the foods.

Technology has been making all manner of products incompatible with our permanent environment, producing a mess from which it may be impossible to escape. Many synthetic materials are creating disposal problems in our society. There are mountains of non-degradable material cluttering and poisoning the landscape. Will imitation protein and amino acids, or what passes for enzymes, likewise leave non-degradable residues when taken inside the human body? The spectator can see the litter of trash on the streets in a slum neighborhood. Little does he suspect that a similar situation may prevail within his own body; that invading trash clogs and pollutes the organs, compounding our health problems.

Our protoplasm has been conditioned by years of development and evolution under conditions as immutable as the Law of Gravity. It has been impregnated with a permanently indelible imprint that is just as distinctive as the trademark stamped on a particular brand of merchandise. It defies duplication by anything science can contrive. Assuming that eventually synthetics that even vaguely resemble amino acids or enzymes will be produced in the laboratory, what are we to do with them? Eat them? Or eat the products resulting from the use of such concoctions in agriculture and animal husbandry? Modern ecology can only say very sternly, "No!" The US Government has been concerned about the problem of preserving food, including meat, particularly for the military. It has been experimenting with giving meat gamma ray treatment to preserve it. These rays are like the type of death-dealing rays atomic bombs give off. Proponents of food radiation claim that the rays go right through the meat and leave no residue. Since nothing *measurable* remains, they boldly proclaim that the meat is wholesome and safe. Steak can be kept on a kitchen shelf at room temperature without spoilage, after being irradiated. Bacteria will have nothing to do with it; they will not attack this ray-embalmed stuff. But there are other factors to consider.

The process of preserving food with dangerous rays has been used on some 20 different foods. Dr. S.A. Goldblith, Department of Nutrition and Food Science, Massachusetts Institute of Technology, wrote in 1966 that the Food and Drug Administration (FDA) had started to issue regulations permitting the sale of radiation-treated foods in the United States. His conclusion about the radiation of food was: "Extensive laboratory data which go far beyond the level of due prudence, have demonstrated the safety of the process and shown that the foods studied can be consumed with impunity." His further remarks show him to be deeply offended that any upstart would be so brazen as to question the safety of irradiated foods after he had put his stamp of approval on them. He was so annoyed he allowed it to spill over on Professor Steward, a British scientist who directed the most damaging experiments which disclosed the possible long-term deleterious effects from consuming irradiated food.

Goldblith stated that his radiated foods had been fed to multiple generations of animals over a 2-year period. But what about after 10 or 20 years? What about the offspring born of mothers in the later period of their reproductive lives (instead of the first offspring of young mothers, as is the usual practice)? Experiments often fail to show up objectionable features of a product unless they are carried out properly and long enough. Considering that hundreds of millions, or even billions of people would be exposed to radiated food, why the rush to endorse it? Let's test it on generations of animals, always taking the last litter of an older female mated with an older male to start members of a new generation. If the first litter of a young female is used, the cumulative effect of harmful inheritance might not be noticeable in a reasonable experimental period. Older parents have a longer exposure to the questionable test material and can pass on more harmful sequelae to future generations. In other words, if one wanted to prove that irradiated foods were completely safe, using young parents would be the method of choice. If the object was to uncover longer-acting mechanisms, however, using older parents would offer a better chance of showing up something in a reasonable length of time.

Using *Drosophila* (the fruit fly) in a research project, a group of scientists at the Indian Agricultural Research Institute in New Delhi (Swaminathan et al., 1963) demonstrated damage to the fly after feeding irradiated food. Their findings have been amplified and confirmed by others. As a result of unfavorable reports questioning the safety of the radiation treatment of food, the FDA reconsidered its former okay of the project. In a report known as the "Status of the Food Irradiation Program," printed by the US Government Printing Office in 1968, the future of rayed food was cast in doubt.

The attack on Professor Steward came as an answer to his paper entitled, "Direct and Indirect Effects of Radiation on Plant Cells: Their Relation to Growth and Growth Induction" (1965). The authors of the report were R.D. Holsten, Ph.D., M. Suggi, Ph.D., and Professor F.C. Steward, F.R.S. (Fellow of the Royal Society). The extensive research was done at the Laboratory of Cell Physiology and Growth, Cornell University. This report stirred up a hornet's nest and caused other investigators to get busy. What Dr. Goldblith didn't like was a part of the summary of the report which stated: "The work has other and obvious implications for the radiation-sterilization of food. If radiation effects may be transmitted to cells via stable radiolysis products derived from sugar, one should clearly know whether or not these have biologically important consequences, both short and long term, before there is widespread use of radiation-sterilized foods that contain sugar." Food sterilization was a pet project of Dr. Goldblith: "The conclusions drawn by Steward et al. are immaterial and unwarranted. It is indeed unfortunate that these conclusions have been given wide publicity by the popular press."

In their report Holsten, Sugii, and Steward brought up the matter of testing the safety of rayed food on fruit flies. They stated there were indications of damage to *Drosophila* which had been reared on an irradiated medium. I agree. Let's forget about rats, mice, rabbits, or guinea pigs for a while, in testing rayed food. They live too long, so it will require a long time to form conclusions—perhaps twenty years. With a concerted effort using the bug variety of subjects, a satisfactory appraisal of the status of rayed food could be achieved perhaps in one or two years. The fruit fly lives out its whole life span in a month or two, compared to a year or two for mice. Working with fruit flies is nothing new to scientists. They have been using them for half a century to test out medical and biological problems. Goldblith said if rayed products damage simple vegetable cells, that proves nothing for higher animals and humans. Quote: "Such effects cannot, however, be compared with defined whole animal systems, such as rats, cats, dogs, chickens and humans, replete with mechanisms for modification, alteration, and digestion of the foods by the alimentary tract and the detoxification and excretion mechanisms of the liver and kidneys."

From this it may be surmised Goldblith does not object to exposing our liver and kidneys to the possibility of some damage from rayed food. In his letter of complaint Goldblith does not mention the fruit fly. The fly is a member of the animal kingdom and is favored with the mechanisms demanded by Goldblith. I do not wish to appear disrespectful to Dr. Goldblith. No doubt he put in a lot of hard work and honest effort on his project. But this matter is far too serious to be passed over lightly. My health has been permanently damaged by a practice formerly in good standing but long since discredited. We have had enough tests on the higher animals. A recent one came out under the heading "The Wholesomeness of Irradiated Mushrooms" (1971), by Van Logten et al. at the Laboratory of Pathology, National Institute of Public Health, The Netherlands. Three generations of rats were reared. The scientists followed the objectionable standard practice of using the first litters to form a new generation, instead of a litter nearing the end of the reproductive life of the parents. No effects attributable to raying were observed on growth, food intake, composition of blood and bone marrow, the activity of certain enzymes, prothrombin time (blood clotting), organ weights, and microscopic analysis of tissue. A clean bill of health. A remarkable confirmation of Goldblith's stand. We surely don't need any more of this kind of rat experiment to prove the safety of rayed food.

Research on food irradiation partially paid for by the US Atomic Energy Commission, Georgia, was conducted by J.H. Brower, E.W. Tilton, and R.R. Cogburn in 1971. They fed the Indian Meal Moth through nine generations on irradiated whole wheat flour and for four generations on raisins treated with gamma rays. There *seemed* to be no harm to the insects or their progeny. But the finding that the females eating the food exposed to the heavier ray dosage produced *more* offspring than those eating normal food raises many questions. What would happen if these insects were fed this rayed food for twenty, fifty, or a hundred generations? The authors themselves stated that the genetic effects of irradiated diets on the fruit fly are controversial.

According to an editorial in *Nature* in 1968, "the Army has its back to the wall on irradiated food." The editors of the journal *Food and Cosmetic Toxicology* (1969) also called attention to the many severe critics of rayed food who point out the possible insults to health resulting from its use. Among findings after more complete studies on animals was the appearance of more tumors in experimental animals using rayed food. It seems that some research people forget to count tumors.

In the *Journal of Agricultural and Food Chemistry* (1970), R.J. Echandi, B.R. Chase, and L.M. Massey, Cornell University, stated that high doses of gamma radiation drastically softened carrots and caused them to leach calcium. J. Seuge, J.L. Morere, and C. Ferradini, Faculté des Sciences, Orsay and Laboratoire Curie, Paris, reported in *Radiation Research* (1971) on feeding gamma-radiated pistachio nuts to Indian Meal Moths, and gamma-radiated potatoes to mealy bugs. The fecundity (power of reproduction) of the Indian Meal Moths was reduced by 32 percent, while the fecundity of mealy bugs was reduced by 41 percent. The authors cite foreign literature claiming that vitamins such as thiamine and ascorbic acid are rather radiosensitive. In spite of this weighty evidence against it, many people of the "today world" are ready to accept food that has been bombarded with dangerous rays with open arms. The editor of the *South African Medical Journal* (1972) wrote a piece entitled "Fresh Meat and Vegetables," in which he pointed out how easy it would be to ship vulnerable fruits to the customer in prime condition after dosing the food with radiation. He said it is not going to be easy to convince the masses that such food is harmless and that it is up to the doctors to do this.

Stop Food Tampering

We need a vigilant public to put an end to food tampering. I have a selfish interest in ray-treated food. I don't want my grandchildren exposed to the stuff. If we don't object, the supermarket shelves will be loaded with it. No refrigeration needed. It will not spoil. Take a piece of rayed meat, put it in a plastic bag to prevent drying out, and place it on a pantry shelf. Examined in a month, it will be as fresh as at the beginning. Normal meat would be putrid with bacteria.

For the business world this innovation is tremendous. It may be impossible for our governing bodies to resist the pressure from business for treatment of food with supervoltage gamma rays; people interested mainly in making money will embrace the method while closing their eyes to treacherous long-term damage. With hindsight, it is hard to forget the positive assurances on the safety of DDT when it first appeared. We were regaled with glorifying stories about its selective activity. DDT would kill only insect pests. It was harmless to the larger animals and man, the popular press broadcast far and wide. The stuff was spread from pole to pole and now resides in the bodies of all creatures, including newborn babies. This is about as comforting as having to carry around a rattlesnake.

If you have followed my line of argument so far you may begin to feel a strong urge to bolster your health by capturing the food enzymes that are to be found in every bit of unheated vegetable or animal matter. Exogenous enzymes are outside your body. They are sociable types. Now let us turn to the more practical matters of the enzyme diet and see how we can invite them in.

6

Making Enzymes
Work for You

THE ENZYME DIET FOR THERAPY
AND NORMAL WEIGHT

Until now we have discussed the evidence for the use of uncooked foods in proper nutrition. But little has been said about the value of uncooked foods in the reversal of problems like obesity and other common health problems, and even less has been said about how you can use specific foods and enzyme supplements to improve your health. In this chapter I will discuss how foods endowed with enzymes normalize body weight, describe their action on glands and the brain, and present an easy way to determine the enzyme content of the different foods available.

THE ENZYME DIET

The Enzyme Diet is a term I have coined to define a regimen in which food is taken uncooked in the raw, unprocessed form, in possession of its full quota of enzymes. Although very few humans can be found who live permanently on this diet, it constitutes the manner of living for all other living organisms. Each species chooses a particular class of substances for sustenance. Although cattle have been known to relish fish, and cats to eat vegetables, each kind of creature has digestive equipment best suited to certain categories of food.

There is a group of persons called "raw fooders" who try to live on a raw diet. In 1912, George A. Drews published a book with the title *Unfired Food and Trophotherapy (Food Cure)*. It consisted mostly of recipes, among them some utilizing ground raw wheat grains. In one of these, ground whole wheat was mixed with honey and flaked nuts and placed in the hot sun to "bake." Although an exceptionally hot sun can mimic a cook stove to a slight extent, the food materials remain mainly raw.

Drews and other raw food eaters advocated the practice because they thought cooking kills the "life principle" in food. They did not know at that time that food contains enzymes and that heat kills them. And it was before the vitamin era. But even without this specific information they were guided by general knowledge of the destructive effect of heat. Likewise, medical literature names many physicians who advocated raw food for curative purposes without understanding the rationale. Without any knowledge of food enzymes, they advocated raw food on a purely empirical basis. There was only one determining factor: results on the patient. Raw foods as therapeutic agents gained popularity in Germany and adjoining countries in the 1920s and 1930s. In 1931, an editorial in the *Journal of the American Medical Association* reviewed the work of three German groups of doctors on raw foods: Loewry and Behrens, Scheunert and Bischoff, and W. Hilsinger. In 1930, the German professor H. Strauss discussed favorably the impact of raw foods in the general scheme of nutrition, reviewing the work of Dr. Max Gerson and Dr. Bircher-Benner. Dr. Gerson's diet in tuberculosis became well known in Germany while he lived there before coming to New York and formulating a nutritional approach to cancer. W. Heupke was another investigator who had numerous reports in German medical journals on the value of raw foods. He claimed that given a meal of raw vegetables, the enzymes of our digestive secretions can penetrate the walls of unruptured plant cells and digest the contents, and then migrate out of the cell through the unbroken wall. He stated that the plant enzymes within the cells assisted the digestion. Heupke published a number of papers in which he detailed experiments to support this position.

RAW MILK DIET

Before the era of pasteurization, the raw milk diet was in vogue and enjoyed acceptance by some physicians. This was in the days when raw milk was for sale in every food store and was delivered by the milkman to the home. Originally milk was not for sale. Every family had cows and produced enough milk, butter, and cheese for its own needs. The cows roamed the pasture and forest to find natural food. They were not fed questionable concentrates to produce more milk. When people began moving to cities, milk became a food of commerce. Cows were bred for large udders to produce more milk. Forcing an animal to produce more milk than necessary for its offspring taxes its economy and increases susceptibility to disease. As a boy, I saw herds needing no veterinarian.

When milk entered commerce, it was handled by many and subject to contamination by bacteria. Mass production resulted in more milk, but the quality suffered. Before the days of refrigeration, cows were kept in large sheds in cities to facilitate prompt delivery to consumers. In some cases, they were kept underground, never seeing sunlight. Tuberculosis became common. Pasteurization was necessary to prevent the spread of communicable disease. It is remarkable that after pasteurization became universal the former therapeutic efficacy of milk was found wanting and milk diets lost their reason for being. Physicians no longer considered milk a remedy. If one wishes to catch a glimpse of what raw milk could do in a variety of ailments there is the book published in 1908 by C.S. Potter, M.D., under the title *Milk Diet as a Remedy for Chronic Disease*. The reader should keep in mind that reference is being made to old-fashioned raw milk with all its enzymes intact. Of course, Dr. Potter knew nothing of food enzymes in milk in 1908. It is important when following any kind of diet to heed advice from a doctor who has experience in that area. In an attempt to cover some highlights on the routine of the raw milk diet, I shall quote a few lines from Dr. Potter's book:

Stout, constipated and toxic individuals must use a fruit diet at least thirty-six hours before the milk diet. The last thousand cases that I have had under observation have averaged about six quarts of milk daily. On an exclusive milk diet, it may be dangerous to take less. Milk is taken every half hour until there have been thirty-two drinks. The minimum time for a milk diet course should be four weeks, which should ordinarily be sufficient to cure any of the following diseases; nervous prostration, general debility, many skin troubles, simple anemia, catarrh, biliousness, constipation, dyspepsia, indigestion, hay fever, piles, insomnia, ulcer of the stomach, malaria, neuralgia, neurasthenia, and the first stages of diseases like consumption, rheumatism, and kidney disease. In more advanced cases longer time is required.

It can be observed that the names given to some of these ailments are not in accord with the present scientific nomenclature. After all,

75 years do make a difference. Also, the word "cure" had a different meaning than the one we use today. It usually meant a course of treatment. That is, people went to hot springs and "took the water cure." I am sure when Dr. Potter put his patients on a raw milk diet he did not realize he was giving them an enzyme treatment. But there can be little doubt that at least 4 weeks of an exclusive raw diet with its full enzyme content must exert a profound influence on anyone's body. Any kind of raw diet cuts down enzyme secretion and gives the enzyme machinery a rest. During my childhood, raw milk was a common daily food. My mother had four quarts of raw milk delivered every day for four of us youngsters. By the time I became interested in raw food in the late 1910s, raw milk was out of the picture. By and large, pasteurization was the law of the land. Therefore, I have had little experience with the raw milk diet as a therapeutic measure. It is still possible to buy raw certified milk in some areas, but it must be pointed out that the customer will very likely not get the same product available in Dr. Potter's day.

In producing commercial raw certified milk, the cows spend their day standing in barns stuffing themselves with an abundance of dry fodder and milk-producing additives. Standardized daily use of penicillin is part of the present operation. The milk cows are denied the right to go on pasture to feed on fresh green vegetation. They are allowed to walk around outside an hour or two in a barren plot for daily exercise. This is a typical factory operation designed for top milk production; the antithesis of milk with full value. The interests of mass production have led to the selection of cows with abnormally large udders. It stands to reason that the so-called "scrub" cows of former times, with their smaller udders and less milk secretion, had less strain on their metabolism and could produce milk of higher health value.

Let us not refer to the amount of fat in milk as the measure of quality, which is established order in the milk industry. To ignore the health intangibles is inexcusable for anyone concerned with human well-being. The full impact of these intangibles can only be appreciated when a comparison is made between the favorable health benefits of raw milk noted by Dr. Potter and his predecessors dating back to the time of Hippocrates, and the negative values of today's pasteurized milk. No one would expect health benefits from an exclusive pasteurized milk diet. It has no medical sponsors or curative value. Medical enthusiasm for milk as a therapeutic agent suffered an abrupt ending with the advent of pasteurization, and its killing of milk enzymes. An important conclusion emerges from studying the long history of milk as a food and as a medicine. When one takes enzymes away from milk, it loses some of its health value and most of its curative properties.

A critical study of the history of use of foods as curative agents forces one to the conclusion that the virtue of effective foods resides in their possessing all of the nutritional factors nature gave them. If something is taken away from a food, such as loss of vitamins, minerals, or enzymes, it becomes an imperfect "minus" food and cannot be expected to carry out the biological traditions of untampered food to maintain a high order of health, let alone cure ailments. The status of raw milk gained as a remedy for chronic diseases throughout hundreds of years vanished with the coming of pasteurized milk. The so-called milk cure, using large quantities of raw milk as an exclusive temporary diet, was practiced formerly as a remedy in many chronic diseases by such physicians as Karrick, Karel, F. von Niemeyer, Winternitz, Potter, and Bremer. Drs. Donkin and Tyson in 1868 advocated seven quarts of raw milk daily for diabetics. This was about 60 years before the insulin era.

Raw milk and its products have a long history of use as foods in Europe, Russia, and the Balkans. These peoples use a great deal of dairy products but diseases of the heart and blood vessels have been comparatively rare. The Danes of a bygone day consumed much raw butter. According to Metchnikoff, many Bulgarian peasants lived a century because they used raw milk and its products lavishly. Why didn't these people suffer from the ravages of cholesterol? Is there something in raw milk and raw butter that makes cholesterol behave? Raw butter seems to be an unusual fat. It looks like we have a situation here pointing to the virtue of the enzymes in raw milk and raw butter in relation to certain diseases, including cardiovascular ailments. Since the milk and fruit juice for sale in these days are not looked upon to cure anything, the results claimed for the same products in the old days can only be ascribed to the presence of food enzymes, while the negative effects of the modern products can be equated with the absence of food enzymes. Vitamins and minerals have remained essentially unchanged in them. If one wished to uphold a position that enzymes in foods are worthless to the living organism, this is only one of the many hurdles it would be necessary to surmount.

Raw Milk Enzymes Alleviate Psoriasis

Some 50 years ago an M.D. in Virginia, Dr. A.B. Grubb, ordered his patients to feast on butter to cure psoriasis (a skin disease). According to modern medical practice, however, fat must be cut down in order to remedy psoriasis. Evidently, Dr. Grubb's butter diet differed in some way from today's fats.

Modern doctors believe that there is a defect in fat utilization in psoriasis patients. In Europe, during World War I, diets lacked fat and oils, and psoriasis became rare. Because there was no indication in Dr. Grubb's report whether or not raw butter was used, I wrote a letter to him dated November 2, 1936, inquiring whether or not raw butter had been used, the amount advised, and the time required to show definite results. Dr. Grubb replied that patients were encouraged to use 2 pounds of butter per week and that raw butter was used in all cases. Patients continued the butter diet for 6 weeks, by which time the psoriasis had improved to an extent to allow the butter ration to be reduced according to the desire of the patient. Dr. Grubb thought the raw butter would soften the skin, but was surprised when the scales diminished. He had no theory to account for the results.

It is known that lipase is one of the principal enzymes in milk and can be expected to be concentrated in raw butter. Since pancreatin (the enzymes secreted by the pancreas, including lipase) has been reported to be of service in the treatment of psoriasis by several dermatologists, it is not inconceivable that Dr. Grubb's good results with raw butter could be ascribed to the intake of large amounts of intact, unextracted lipase. There are indications in the literature that enzymes ingested with their natural substrates perform better in the digestive tract and do not suffer in the same degree from exposure to its hazards as does pancreatin. If the lipase of raw butter or the lipase of pancreatin or other exogenous enzymes is to be of service in instances where the pancreatic secretion is not impaired, the digestion should take place in the gastric fundus during the period of digestive inertia. Experience has shown that enteric-coated enzymes are ineffective in psoriasis.

ENZYME DEFICIENCY DISEASE

Some doctors have noted good results when enzymes were used by the patient afflicted with psoriasis. Lipase, which is an ingredient in the enzyme formula, was singled out for special emphasis. Lipase is also found in raw butter. Those doctors getting the best results emphasized one point strongly; massive dosage for many months is required. Dr. L.N. Elson (1935), a dermatologist of New Orleans, Louisiana, says this about psoriasis: "Psoriasis belongs to a class of enzyme deficiency diseases. Massive doses of pancreas extract will cure it." A teaspoonful of pancreas enzyme powder in connection with meals 3 times each day, which is 3 times the usual dose, is advised by the doctor. Dr. J. Sellei (1937), Chief Dermatologist, Hungarian State Railway Hospital, Budapest, believed many forms of skin ailments are due to enzyme derangements in the stomach, duodenum, pancreas, or liver. His treatment included daily use of 3 to 5 ounces of raw pancreas and the same amount of raw liver. These were minced and blended with juice or soup and eaten raw. He also recommended 8 to 10 pancreatin tablets (not enteric-coated) and 4 or 5 liver tablets daily, one hour before meals. Dr. Sellei stressed that these measures must be continued for many months, otherwise no satisfactory results can be expected. Where large amounts of concentrated enzymes are to be used, it is essential that the patient be observed by a doctor with experience along these lines.

How Enzyme Tablets Work

Two dermatologists, Drs. E.M. Farber and H.M. Schneidman (1957), gave 36 psoriasis patients from 3 to 9 pancreatin enzyme tablets daily for 6 to 18 weeks. They reported poor results. They sent a questionnaire to dermatologists and received a reply from 28 who had used enzymes to treat psoriasis. Twenty-four of them reported no improvement, and 4 reported minimal improvement. In recent years enteric-coated tablets have been employed, whereas in former times the enzymes were used in powder form or in tablets with a plain coating. Enteric tablets are so named because they will not dissolve in the acid stomach, but only become active in the alkaline juices of the intestine ("enteric" means "in the intestine"). When the food and tablets reach the intestine, the pancreas pours its alkaline enzyme juice on them. By the time the coated tablets are dissolved and ready to work, they may not be needed. The enzymes of the pancreatic juice usually digest all the food promptly except in those few cases where the secretion is deficient.

It is only when the pancreas is on strike that enteric-coated enzymes are superior to plain enzymes and can help out. Otherwise, enzymes active in the fundus of the stomch are preferred. They do work before stomach acid becomes too strong. There is evidence that highly purified enzymes are less resistant to the action of gastric juice than food enzymes which are protected by their own food substrates. This may be why some doctors can report results while others have no results. It may depend on the kind of enzymes employed. Crude enzymes such as lipase of raw butter and lipase of whole pancreas can function in the non-glandular stomach fundus and are better protected from hostile elements in the stomach and intestine.

FOOD AND GLAND SIZE

Previously, food was considered to have no effects except for the production of heat and energy from fats and carbohydrates and the repair of tissues by proteins. Now it is known that food can change organs and tissues, including glands, for either better or worse. The fact that food can change the size and weight of these important glands (pituitary, testicle, ovary, pancreas, adrenal, thyroid) has been demonstrated over and over again by careful experimenters during past years. Professor Jackson and co-workers at the University of Minnesota fed white rats a diet containing 80 percent sugar (enzyme-free) and reported marked differences in the size and weight of all principal organs and glands. The importance of the pituitary in nature's scheme may be guessed by its being doubly shielded from physical injury, first by a substantial bony skull and then by being buried in the recesses of the brain. Since the pituitary gland has importance as a body regulator, the influence of food in modifying its size and function merits special attention. The pituitary has been credited with being a "master gland" of the body by virtue of exercising control and coordination of other endocrine glands. It has a degree of control out of proportion to its size.

Adverse Effects of Dextrose on Pituitary and Pancreas

Drs. H.R. Jacobs and A.R. Colwell of the University of Chicago exposed 20 dogs to continuous intravenous administration of dextrose until the animals died, which was from one to seven days. Examination of the organs after death showed specific intense hemorrhage into and the destruction of the pancreas and anterior lobe of the pituitary, while the other organs were fairly normal, except the liver, which was much enlarged. The authors remarked in their report in 1936 that dextrose imposes a great strain upon the metabolism. We might add that the results also hint at the possible gland damage produced by the one-third pound of refined sugar each person consumes every day. Perhaps the only reason we have not heard more about the mischief caused by dextrose in the living body is that less of it is used in human diets. But dextrose is also responsible for producing physiological changes when fed as the source of carbohydrate in laboratory diets in research on various projects. Tests have shown it stimulates the secretion of uncalled-for enzymes.

Dr. A Schonemann, a German pathologist, examined a total of 111 human pituitary glands. In his report of 1892, he found the percentage of abnormal glands (the weight of a gland was used as a measure of its normality) in persons dying of various diseases and old age as follows:

Table 6.1
ABNORMAL PITUITARIES AND AGE

Age	% Abnormal
Newborn	27
1 year to 20 years	50
20 years to 40 years	71
40 years to 60 years	90
Over 60 years	100

The finding of abnormal glands in 27 percent of newly born dead babies supports the contention that the diet of the mother has far-reaching effects on her unborn child.

Dr. A.T. Rasmussen (1924), Department of Anatomy, University of Minnesota, quoted Dr. Comte (1898), who examined 39 pituitary glands from persons 21 to 70 years of age. He reflects the same idea about the increasing abnormality of the pituitary with increasing age as Schonemann; no human pituitary after the age of 50 is normal. In a dissertation on the normal and pathological anatomy of the human pituitary, H. Creutzfeld (1909), also quoted by Rasmussen, reported on the examination of 110 cases. He concluded the gland gets bigger until age 30 and starts losing weight after 50 years of age. More recent information (1965), from autopsy studies in adult men, shows unimpressive effects of age on the relative weight of the pituitary. However, according to Finch and Hayflick in the *Handbook of the Biology of Aging* (1977), microscopic changes in the human pituitary gland during adult aging include decreased vascularity, increased connective tissue, and a change in the distribution of cell types.

The finding that perhaps all or nearly all persons over 60 have abnormal pituitary glands should provide a rude awakening to the constancy of a biological law that proclaims that we cannot steal from nature and get away with it. Nature is a relentless accountant. Her records are indelibly etched into the protoplasm of our tissues.

Heat-treated, enzyme-free, refined items of food caused the most drastic deviations in pituitary gland size and appearance. When animals were fed diets greatly restricted in enzymes, the damage in the pituitary was identical or similar to that found in human beings subsisting on conventional food with greatly lowered food enzyme intake. This finding was confirmed by examination of animal tissues. The intimate relation of the endocrine glands and enzymes is shown when surgical removal of some of the glands leads to pronounced change in the enzyme level of the blood. A similar change occurs when the endocrine balance is disturbed by injecting gland extracts, disclosing a sensitive interdependence between enzymes and endocrine glands. Hormones influence the activity of enzymes, and enzymes are necessary in the formation of hormones. These facts have been unearthed only after a great deal of research by many independent scientific workers and carry a message of profound importance.

Glands Influence Obesity

The idea that overactive or underactive glands can influence body weight is not new. A reducing method which has lost some of its original popularity involves the use of thyroxin, an extract made from the thyroid glands of animals and put into a tablet. When physicians prescribe thyroxin by mouth to lose weight, the heart races, the victim loses weight, the nervous system is keyed up, and the eyes bulge. In this way, fat is burned. If too large a dose is used, or if the drug is taken over a longer period, the patient may develop the condition known as nervousness or anxiety.

However, the concept that an individual has the power to influence his overactive glands has never been presented before to my knowledge. A person desiring to shed surplus weight can do so, and can also keep it off. The first thing a weight reducer must do is capture the idea that certain foods excite and whip up the glands that control obesity. If you cease whipping a galloping horse, he will slow down. If you stop whipping the glands, they go more slowly, and excess weight starts diminishing. According to the work of Drs. Jacobs and Colwell, cited above, the pituitary and pancreas get some of the whipping. Their excess secretions have abnormal repercussions on other endocrine glands, and diseases are born. If you would do almost anything to reduce, but cannot tolerate the idea of being confronted with a lot of technical terminology, the following discussion of raw calories and cooked calories may be just what you need. The *kind* of calories that are used is just as important as *how many*.

SECRETS OF WEIGHT REDUCTION

The calorie lists in use make no distinction between raw calories and cooked calories. This is, in my opinion, a very serious oversight. I can find no indication in scientific literature presenting the idea that raw food is inherently less fattening than the same amount of calories in cooked food, and that cooked food overstimulates the endocrine system. The quick rejoinder from some critics will be that less raw food is assimilated. That may be precisely true. Or, put another way, too much fat-inducing cooked food is assimilated. If enough raw food is absorbed to promote normal weight, this can be accepted as the ideal function of food. If the same amount of cooked food brings on overweight, the cooked calories must give an accounting of their bizarre conduct. It makes good logic to remember that the vast multitudes of creation have been thriving on raw food, but not getting fat, for millions of years. Raw calories are relatively non-stimulating to glands and tend to stabilize weight. Cooked calories excite glands and tend to be fattening. I am not here referring to something like a dish of cooked spinach, which has few calories in the first place. But a slice of bread or a boiled potato stimulates glands and will put on the ounces which add up into many pounds. Let us learn something from animals. Technical men in the business of extracting the maximum profit from farm animals found it was not economical to feed hogs raw potatoes. The hogs would not get fat enough. Cooking the potatoes, however, produced the fat hogs that brought the farmer the kind of money required to make a profit. This in spite of the extra expense of labor and energy involved in cooking!

Raw Versus Cooked Calories

As a general rule we may say a raw potato is not as fattening as the same potato cooked. A raw banana is not as fattening as a baked banana. A raw apple is not as fattening as a baked apple. A spoonful of raw honey is not as fattening as the same amount of calories in the form of white sugar. Two ounces of raw walnuts are less fattening than the same amount of roasted walnuts. A glass of raw (freshly squeezed) fruit juice should put on less weight than a glass of ready-made juice.

There is no direct experimental evidence to support many of these statements relative to raw and cooked calories. But there are a great many related facts, originating in research laboratories scattered over the world, which coalesce to support the doctrine. During some 40 years I have been actively engaged in library research; collecting, cataloguing, and trying to evaluate data from these sources that comprise the substance of this manuscript. Laboratory rats and mice are used for many types of studies. In many cases the period of observation may be only a few weeks, or possibly 2 or 3 months. During this short period the animals are fed the standard "scientific" manufactured chow diet, but no indications develop that the diet is not effective in preventing obesity or the onset of disease. Some, but not many, studies require prolonged observation of animals exposed to the chow diet for 1 or 2 years and it is here that obesity and disease show up. The chow diet may be considered to be roughly equivalent to the average human diet. While it has nothing raw, it contains more vitamins and minerals than the food consumed by many humans. Therefore, if the chow diet induces obesity and a multitude of diseases in laboratory animals, its equivalent can be expected to do the same in man.

Some intriguing experiments were performed on normal people and diabetics by Drs. S.M. Rosenthal and E.E. Ziegler at George Washington University Hospital in 1929. The subjects ate almost two ounces of raw starch and then had blood tests for sugar. Eating cooked starch, as is well known, causes the blood sugar of diabetics to skyrocket, unless they use insulin. The diabetics in this study used no insulin and yet after raw starch ingestion, the blood sugar rose only 6 milligrams the first half hour. Then it decreased 9 milligrams after 1 hour, and 14 milligrams 2½ hours after ingestion of the raw starch. In some diabetic individuals, the decrease in blood sugar was as much as 35 milligrams. In the normal persons there was a slight increase followed by a slight decrease in blood sugar in 1 hour. This is convincing evidence that there is a difference between raw and cooked calories.

Raw Fat Is Not Fattening

A pound of raw beefsteak may add only protein to the tissues and not put on any fat. On the other hand, the same amount of cooked beefsteak may give the eater a little unwanted fat. Many peoples, such as the primitive, isolated Eskimo, as we have seen, ate raw meat as a part of their diet. Dr. V.E. Levine of Omaha, Nebraska, examined 3,000 primitive Eskimos during 3 trips to the Arctic and found only one overweight person. These Eskimos ate enormous amounts of fat. It is hard to escape the conclusion that raw food is not fattening in the conventional sense. Raw blubber and other fats used by the Eskimo, along with the raw butter that was formerly enjoyed throughout America, do not promote weight gain. Raw fats evidently belong in a special pigeonhole in nutritional speculations. Furthermore, medical reports on primitive, isolated Eskimos emphasize that these heavy eaters of raw animal fat had no hypertension (high blood pressure) or hardening of the arteries. All raw fats are inhabited by the enzyme lipase which should not be ignored in speculations on a perfect diet. This enzyme is absent in the kind of fats presently used in the kitchen.

Nice Calories and Evil Ones

Avocados are blessed with a lot of nice calories. Ever hear of anyone getting fat on them? Or on bananas, which also have plenty of raw calories? It would be an exceptional person who could eat enough bananas to get fat. All of these high-calorie raw foods might fill out a thin individual to a slight degree, but they know just where to put the ounces, and when to stop. They will not drape the weight about in ugly disarray over the exterior, or clog up delicate heart arteries. The doctor who invented the banana diet for reducing, George Harrop, put his overweight patients on a milk and banana diet and wrote up his results in the *Journal of the American Medical Association* in 1934. His results should dispose of the idea that bananas are fattening because their calories count up to so-and-so. To judge a banana, an avocado, an apple, or an orange by its calories is just as misleading and false as evaluating the moral stature of a pretty woman by her exterior embellishments. There is a difference between raw and cooked calories.

OTHER FACTS PERTINENT TO WEIGHT REDUCTION

Some light on the way in which the brain can control the appetite for better or for worse was supplied by scientists at the University of Western Ontario, Canada. They inserted electrodes into the brains of 33 rats in an area called the hypothalamus. By using a weak electric current to stimulate the hypothalamus, the investigators could make the rats eat or drink more or less at will. I have a theory that the same area of the brain is being constantly bombarded in stout people by certain chemical agents floating around in the bloodstream looking for ways to create mischief. It is suspected these stimulants are produced by the highly refined carbohydrate materials commonly eaten. This piece of research was performed by G.L. Mogenson, C.G. Gentil, and A.F. Stevenson (1971).

A doctor at Columbia University, B.N. Berg, wanted to learn if the amount of food eaten had anything to do with health. He reported in 1960 that 339 rats were used to test out this idea. Some of them were permitted to eat all they wished, while others were given only measured amounts of food. When they were about 800 days old the restricted rats weighed about 40 percent less than the unrestricted. Restricted rats had smooth, clean fur and fine hair. Their teeth showed no abnormalities. They were lively and aggressive and consumed the food promptly. On autopsy there was little or no evidence of body fat. In contrast with the sleek appearance of restricted rats, the coat of the unrestricted feeders was coarse and soiled. The incisor teeth were elongated and frequently fractured. They became sluggish, slept most of the time, accepting food pellets but storing them away without eating them. Examination at autopsy revealed large deposits of fat which accounted for most of the difference in weight between the two groups. Female fertility was better in the animals eating less. The regular stock diet was used for all animals. This consisted of manufactured pellets of processed, heat-treated food, suitably supplemented with commercial vitamins and minerals. Whether animals would react in the same way if the experiment had utilized a raw diet is not known, since it has not been tried, according to my information. However, wild animals eat all they wish of natural, raw food and remain in fine physical condition.

Anatomists have learned that as the young organism grows, the weight of its organs assumes a progressively smaller portion of the total body weight. This is true of the pancreas, kidneys, heart, brain, etc. But the fat accumulation behaves in a directly contrary manner, at least in response to a heat-treated diet. Fat becomes a progressively larger share of the total body weight as growth continues to maturity. This is shown in Table 6.2. The figures on the rat are from V. Korenchevsky, Lister Institute, London, *The Journal of Pathology and Bacteriology* 54:13-24 (1942). The figures on the goose are from R.H. Roberson and D.W. Francis, New Mexico State University, *Poultry Science* 44:835-9 (1965). Abdominal fat weights are expressed here as grams per 100 grams of body weight.

Table 6.2

AMOUNT OF ABDOMINAL FAT ACCORDING TO
AGE AND BODY WEIGHT

Average Data on 509 Normal Rats			Average Data on 45 Male White Chinese Geese		
Age Days	Body Weight Grams	Abdominal Fat %	Age Weeks	Body Weight Grams	Abdominal Fat %
25	63	0.88	4	1480	0.98
35	97	1.36	8	2968	1.92
45	174	2.80	10	3272	1.87
55	210	3.78	12	4193	2.21
65	256	4.87	14	4630	2.49
85	297	6.70	16	5042	3.22
113	311	6.54	18	4642	3.71
175	441	8.20	20	4315	3.55
350	523	9.82	22	4900	3.73
450	536	8.00			

During the time the body weight of the goose was increasing about 3 or 4 times, the abdominal fat was multiplying more than 10 times. In the rat, between ages 25 days and 450 days, body weight increased from 63 grams to 536 grams, or 8 times, and abdominal fat increased from 0.554 to 42.9 grams, or 75 times. Stored fat is nature's device to guard against starvation in the event food is unavailable for long periods. For wild creatures this is the mechanism for maintaining life under adverse conditions. But such acute scarcity of calories is seldom a human problem in the Western world. Refrigerators and warehouses have taken over the job of food storage and made it unnecessary for man to carry a supply of reserve calories under his skin.

Doctors at Harvard Medical School discovered how to make mice fat. There were 3 groups. One group was made fat by injection of a chemical called gold thioglucose which made a lesion in a particular area of the brain. In another group a lesion was placed in the same area by surgical means. The third group inherited a tendency toward fatness. What went on secretively inside the body was worse than that which transpires within the smoke-filled rooms of a partisan political caucus. The body weight doubled. The liver became twice as heavy in some animals. There was an enlargement of the heart and some increase in the kidneys and pancreas. The only parts becoming smaller in the fat mice were the brains in all of them and sex organs in some. These investigations were made by Drs. N.B. Marshall, S.B. Andrus, and J. Mayer and reported in 1957.

Why Some People Have Trouble Losing Weight

Dr. G.E. Burch, of the Department of Medicine, Tulane University, has a new idea on the genesis of obesity. It was written up in the *American Heart Journal* in 1971. This brand new wrinkle can show the overweight individual what makes it so tough sometimes to shed pounds. Understanding the mechanics of the process can put new resolve into the determination to diet. Dr. Burch has shown that if animals are overfed after birth their fat cells multipy faster than normally. Once growth and cell proliferation cease, the number of fat cells is constant throughout the remainder of life. The voracious infant eater can reach adulthood with more than 3 times as many fat cells as a normal eater! If a person with a normal number of fat cells stuffs them full of fat by hearty eating, it will show up only as plumpness. But an individual with 3 times as many fat cells, eating the same amount of food, has 3 times as much room to store fat. If each cell is filled, obesity results. And such an individual must show 3 times as much vigilance at the dinner table to keep the army of fat cells only one-third full and remain just pleasantly plump. It pays to remember that one can stuff on raw food with little danger of producing excess weight, providing it is eaten in place of other food, and not in addition to it.

The Value of Avoiding Frequent Snacks

Two rat experiments carried out independently throw some light on the possible effects snacking and frequent eating versus restricted feeding for a 2-hour daily period have on body weight and lifespan. Two separate groups of researchers participated: G.A. Leveille, University of Illinois (1972) and G. Pose, P. Fabry and H.A. Ketz, Institute Ernahrung, Potsdam, Germany (*Nutritional Abstracts and Reviews* 38:7027, 1968). Both groups found that the rats fed but once a day had a lower body weight and higher enzyme activities in the pancreas and fat cells. Leveille also found that the lifespan of the controlled eaters was longer by 17 percent.

The above American and German research has shown more enzymes were found in the pancreas and other tissues after eating a solitary daily meal than when the animals were permitted to eat at will throughout the day. But we must not forget that all of these experimental results are based on the use of 100 percent heat-treated, enzyme-free laboratory diets. Such experiments with raw food are as scarce as the proverbial hen's teeth. Nevertheless, it is clear that heat-treated food acts as a powerful stimulus for enzyme production by the body. If the enzymes are manufactured only once each day, there will not be as many of them used up as when food is eaten, and enzymes are produced, 5 or 10 times each day. Perhaps that is the reason more enzymes are found in the tissues following a single daily feeding and why these animals live longer (688 days against 587 days). Science has no idea how long human beings could live if their tissues never suffered the chemical abuse of unnatural food. Eighty years might just be a starter.

Tissue Enzymes Die Out

Leveille also discovered that the enzyme activities in the tissues became weaker as the rats got older, so that at the age of 18 months (old age for the rats on the modern enzyme-free fabricated diets) the enzymes were much weaker than in the young rat. For instance, he represented the activity of a certain tissue enzyme in rats 1 month of age by 1040 units, while in rats 18 months old this value had shrunken to 184 units. This is in line with older scientific data testifying to the decrease of enzyme activity of the tissues and fluids of insects, animals, and humans as old age arrrives. Some of the older experiments along this line were presented in my volume, *The Status of Food Enzymes in Digestion and Metabolism* (1946), which is available in some of the technical libraries. The book was reprinted under the title *Food Enzymes for Health and Longevity* in 1980.

It can be accepted as a working rule that the enzyme potential is limited and withers as time marches on. The more lavishly a young body gives up its enzymes, the sooner the state of enzyme poverty, or old age, is reached. As a test for enzyme sufficiency, it is not enough to examine some of the digestive secretions, although these have shown less enzyme activity in later life. More important is the status of intracellular or tissue enzymes.

Reducing While Asleep

Animals have a secret about reducing. They just go to sleep. It's as easy as that. No arduous exercises at all. There are creatures that lose weight while sleeping. It is called hibernation, the winter sleep of animals. There is also a summer sleep known as estivation. The winter sleepers get fattened up before winter sets in. Then they curl up in a secluded spot and let the months go by. In the meantime, the only part of the sleepers not taking it easy is their fat-burning enzymes. They keep busy dissolving just enough of the fat store to keep the temperature of the body a little above freezing. Just enough fat is burned to keep the heart beating ever so feebly and the respiration so sluggish as to be imperceptible. When the warmth of spring awakens the once-fat sleeper, the excess of fat has vanished. A tiny animal may lose only ounces, but a bear might lose 50 pounds of fat. These animals eat raw diets and have no fear of enzyme deficiencies. That's the key to their weight loss.

But there is a hint that some extremely overweight people may be short of certain enzymes. In 1966, Dr. David Galton of the Tufts University School of Medicine, made some tests on the abdominal fat of 11 extra heavyweights (ranging from 280 to 430 pounds, with an average of 340 pounds) and found an enzyme deficiency in their fat deposits. Lipase is the enzyme found to be deficient in obese humans. It can be said that lipase is involved in some way with fat metabolism. It may be that obesity and abnormal cholesterol deposits both have their genesis in our failure to permit fat predigestion in the upper stomach (food-enzyme stomach) by destroying the natural lipase content of fatty foods.

ENZYME DIET FOODS

At this point it is opportune to consider how to balance a diet containing cooked food and raw food if one wishes to replace the enzymes missing in the cooked portion. Raw vegetables in the form of salads and fruit are the kinds of raw food used by most people. While these low-calorie foods have some enzymes, they are more useful for their vitamin and mineral content. High-calorie foods have far more of the 3 main digestive enzymes, but unfortunately these foods are customarily eaten cooked and hence without enzymes.

With a meal of meat, potatoes, and bread, many people include a combination vegetable salad. This will not provide enough food enzymes, although every little bit helps. Foods with a high calorie content, such as meat, potatoes, and bread also have high enzyme values when they are raw. When these foods are eaten as served at the table they are enzymeless and cannot be balanced with salad vegetables, which can give you an abundance of minerals and vitamins, but not enzymes.

Some foods which are endowed with both calories and enzymes are palatable in the raw state and some are not. Examples of the former are bananas, avocados, grapes, mangoes, olives from the tree, fresh raw dates, fresh raw figs, raw honey, raw butter, and unpasteurized milk; germinated, inhibitor-free raw cereal grains and seeds; and germinated, inhibitor-free raw tree nuts. If commerce could supply these foods in the raw state, such a diet could offer high-quality proteins, fats, and carbohydrates, and with the addition of salad vegetables, it would fill our nutritional needs.

I have stated earlier that a diet containing 75 percent of raw calories and 25 percent of cooked calories is a vast improvement over the virtually enzymeless diet used by most people. The foods I singled out above are moderately endowed with both food enzymes and calories and can be eaten along with other raw salad vegetables, sprouts, greens, and cooked food to supply all the bodily nutritional requirements.

SUPPLEMENTAL FOOD ENZYMES

In our dialogue I have mentioned supplemental enzymes. Let us discuss this aspect of the enzyme subject. One of the first enzyme supplements used by doctors was pepsin, prepared from the stomachs of pigs. It was used for patients whose digestion of protein was impaired, required a highly acid medium to do its work, and would not work on fats and carbohydrates. Another enzyme supplement is made from the pancreas from slaughterhouse animals. Its enzymes digest proteins, fats, and carbohydrates. The fault with pancreas extract is that its enzymes work best in neutral or slightly alkaline media. Its home is the alkaline duodenum. Pepsin is at home in the stomach because gastric juice is highly acid due to the presence of hydrocholoric acid. Pancreatic enzymes are normally secreted and flow into the alkaline intestine and will not work in acid.

In order to make pancreatic extract suitable for oral use it is made into tablets covered with a so-called enteric coating. This prevents the tablets from dissolving in the acid stomach. But when they reach the intestine the alkaline juice dissolves the coating and releases the enzymes. The purpose of these pancreatic tablets is to promote digestion of food in cases where the pancreas fails to make these enzymes. But hyposecretion of the pancreas is rare. As I have pointed out, the pancreas and other organs secreting digestive enzymes make far too many enzymes because we fail to put food enzymes into the stomach to predigest our food. Because the pancreatic tablets cannot perform predigestion, there is little need for them.

I first became aware of enzymes in foods in 1932. At that time pancreatic extract was frequently used in powder form. But I soon realized that what was needed was an enzyme extract which could digest in mild acid. This would permit predigestion of food in the upper stomach before the stomach acid became too strong. The enzymes of many foods, from both meat and plants, can operate in mild acid, but the cost of extracting these food enzymes is prohibitive. Certain industries also had need for enzymes that would digest in acid media, for example, to aid the removal of starch in de-sizing textiles and in separating protein fragments from hides. The Chinese and Japanese originally found that fungi were good producers of acid enzymes and that extracts of various enzymes could be pepared from them. I formulated a compound embodying the three major enzymes, protease, amylase, and lipase, which digest protein, starch, and fat, respectively.

Fungi have been used in China and other Oriental countries for thousands of years in preparing various foods, many derived from soybean. Fungi called *Aspergilli* supplied the enzymes for making tasty and easily digested food products from soybeans. Japan is far ahead of us in producing enzymes from *Aspergillus oryzae* and other wholesome fungi, supplying enzymes for digesting proteins, carbohydrates, and fats. Yeast and mushrooms are fungi. There are hundreds of varieties of *Aspergilli*, a few of which produce aflatoxins and are not wholesome. Experienced people use only the wholesome varieties.

To obtain the desired enzymes, a selected strain of wholesome *Aspergillus oryzae* is cultured on food materials such as wheat bran, or soybeans to which various minerals have been added. Different combinations of various food substrates produce the several enzymes needed, such as amylase, protease, and lipase. Extracts of these enzymes are dried into powders and put into capsules. The *Aspergillus* enzymes are especially valuable for gastric predigestion because they digest best in mild acid, while the pancreatic and salivary enzymes digest in neutral and alkaline media. *Aspergillus* enzyme supplements and food enzymes both work in the mild acid media that are found in the stomach one half to one hour after food is eaten.

For most effective predigestion, the enzyme capsule should be taken with the meal. If you wait until finishing the meal, you delay action of the enzymes. I chew an enzyme capsule with my food because I wish to start the digestive process immediately. When raw food is chewed, the enzymes in it are released and its digestion begins instantly, even before the food is swallowed. The same thing happens when an enzyme capsule is chewed with your food. Some might find the taste of the enzyme powder objectionable but if you swallow the capsule without chewing it, time is required for it to dissolve and release its enzymes. Some people open the capsule instead and sprinkle the enzyme powder on the food. If you happen to have some coated enzyme tablets, or enzyme capsules containing bile, do not chew them. They are very bitter. Coated tablets are not intended for predigesting food in the stomach. You would be wasting your money if you bought them for predigestion, for they do not dissolve in the food-enzyme stomach, but later, in the small intestine.

ENZYME THERAPY

Can you treat yourself with concentrated enzyme supplements for various ailments? Generally, no. It requires specialized knowledge and experience. Success with therapy in established diseases usually involves massive or frequent dosages or both, and is strictly a job for a doctor. Moreover, if the full potentiality of enzyme therapy is to be realized in cases of advanced, serious disease, a course of proper enzyme therapy must be carried out in a hospital or other institution having adequate nursing facilities. In many cases, part of the program utilizes a special diet, tailored to the case. Multiple small feedings of food throughout the day may be indicated, each feeding coupled with the ingestion of the enzymes. Many years ago, I spent about ten years as a member of a sanitarium staff where special diet procedures were employed in the management of a wide range of chronic and intractable diseases. I therefore am in a position to appreciate the profound impact an amalgamation of specialized dietary therapy and intensive enzyme therapy could have on these human ailments.

It is illogical to expect a full treatment program to be carried out at home with the precision and detail required. One or two units, usually capsules, at a meal is adequate to assist predigestion in the food-enzyme stomach. This is a nutritional supplementation. You are replacing enzymes which are supposed to be in your food, but are not. The amount used as a nutritional supplement is not sufficient for therapeutic use in many intractable states, especially where the patient wants to see results as soon as possible. Using more units requires careful professional supervision, possibly for prolonged periods.

7

Little Known Facts About Raw Foods

ENZYME INHIBITORS

I have already singled out some palatable foods moderately endowed with both calories and enzymes, such as raw milk and butter, honey, banana, fig, date, avocado, grape, and mango. Tree nuts and other palatable seeds, beans, and grains contain superb protein and fat intended by nature for the perpetuation of their own species. To fulfill this duty, seeds must be endowed with a relatively rich enzyme heritage, far more than other parts such as leaves. But because enzymes are restless, active entities, nature had to put a rein on them and make them dormant until such a time as the seed could fall to the ground and be adequately covered with soil. These reins are called enzyme inhibitors and are inactivated by the seed's enzymes when moisture from rain is absorbed by the seed as it finds a suitable niche in soil and begins germinating (sprouting) to form a seedling.

It is obvious that enzyme inhibitors are needed only in the seeds and not in other parts of a plant. But what is required for the well-being of seeds poses problems for animals and humans wanting to eat the seeds for food. In 1944, enzyme inhibitors in seeds were discovered independently by E.D. Bowman, Indiana University, and W.E. Ham and R.M. Sandstedt, Nebraska Agricultural Experiment Station. Prior to that (approximately 1920 to 1940), scores of chemists referred to "free" and "bound" enzymes in seeds, but did not understand the mechanism of inhibition. It was known that the addition of protein-digesting enzymes to seeds would free their enzymes from the bondage and increase enzyme activity greatly. Germination did the same thing. Later it was found out that the added enzymes inactivated the in-

119

hibitors and in that way increased enzyme activity. It was also determined that germination (sprouting) of seeds neutralizes or inactivates enzyme inhibitors. Another point I must bring out is that enzyme activity in the *seed* is at its height when the sprout is approximately ¼-inch long, whereas very little enzyme activity is found in the *sprout*. As the sprout grows longer during the germination process, enzyme activity in the seed weakens, but we do not know if enzymes increase in the sprout at the same time. When I was making such tests many years ago it did not occur to me to make this one, and I have never found a report of others doing such research.

The foregoing information is useful as a guide to the use of tree nuts as food. If you eat substantial quantities of raw pecans, walnuts, Brazil nuts, filberts, or others, you have a choice of swallowing enzyme capsules with them to neutralize their enzyme inhibitors, or first germinating the nuts and letting nature do the job through the increased enzyme activity resulting from germination. In the forest, squirrels make a practice of burying nuts in the ground and digging them up for food after they have germinated. Many years ago I fed squirrels pecans near my home. Sometimes they would break the shells and eat the nuts. But more often they would bury the nuts. Weeks or months later I would find empty holes where they had buried their hoard. They evidently are guided by the odor of the germinated nuts in locating them. But they fail in some instances and a seedling grows. This type of symbiotic behavior is part of nature's scheme. The squirrel must bury nuts to get the germinated victuals it needs. The tree is glad to give the squirrel this food in return for the squirrel's labor in burying nuts, some of which grow into trees.

The periodic scientific literature is teeming with data about the damage a diet including large quantities of enzyme inhibitors can do to growing chickens and rats. Such a diet includes large quantities of raw soybeans. Cooking the soybeans destroys the inhibitors, but it also does away with the enzymes. When similar diets were fed to adult dogs, the harm from the inhibitors seemed to be masked. From this we could jump to the unwarranted conclusion that enzyme inhibitors are harmless to adult humans, but my personal experiences indicate otherwise.

PERSONAL EXPERIENCES

Let me tell you about some personal experiences with enzyme inhibitors. In the year 1918 or thereabouts, I was imbued with the idea of trying to avoid cooked food because of the potential destructiveness of heat. The length of the intestinal tract in humans is about twelve times that of the trunk, while in carnivorous animals, such as lions and tigers, it is only three or four times the length of the trunk. From this I can draw the conclusion that one reason for a shorter intestine in carnivora is to more rapidly dispose of a highly putrefactive diet. There certainly must be other reasons. Since carnivora have a much shorter intestinal tract than humans, I thought that raw meat was unsuited for the human diet and that the protein and fat of palatable raw tree nuts would take its place. As near as I can remember, after a period of about two months during which I consumed liberal quantities of raw tree nuts of several kinds, I began experiencing an unpleasant heavy sensation in the abdomen, and a feeling of extreme fullness, and some nausea. The symptoms were pronounced enough to force my giving up this tasty diet. Almost anyone can eat several nuts without feeling any effect. But it is common knowledge that nuts "are heavy on the stomach" if consumed in substantial quantity. The enzyme inhibitors in seeds explain the mystery, but they were not identified until 1944.

In 1932, when I discovered food enzymes, I counted myself with the very few in believing we possessed the last and final revelations in nutritional knowledge. Vitamins were rapidly gaining recognition as important nutritonal factors, and minerals were getting some dignity after their long and ignoble status as "ash." Imagine my shock and dismay in 1932 when I was confronted with reports from commercial chemists complaining that enzymes were causing problems such as color changes in some frozen vegetables. The chemists decided that the solution was to destroy the enzymes by heat, since they knew nothing about the nutritional value of food enzymes, and were concerned only about the salability of the product. Upon reflection, it becomes obvious that enzymes exist in all living things and become food enzymes when the food is eaten. But until I found out how ultrasensitive enzymes are to heat, I did not realize that the human race had been trying to get along without a whole category of food ingredients since cooking began. Therefore, instead of 1932 being an era representing a pinnacle in nutritional knowledge, I have come to regard it as the dark ages of nutrition.

Upon becoming food-enzyme-conscious I was more concerned than ever with trying to eat as much raw food as possible. The experience with nuts caused me to virtually leave them out of the diet. But when General Mills Corporation initiated a program of supplying freshly milled raw wheat germ to the public by mail, I subscribed to the service. Wheat germ had been shown to be an excellent source of the B vitamins. But I also knew that it contained various enzymes in a more concentrated form than in other foods. What I did not know in 1935 was that raw wheat germ was also loaded with enzyme inhibitors, which were not discovered until the year 1944. At any rate, I began displacing my breakfast cereal with an equal serving of raw wheat germ. The product was rather palatable, but such a large serving is far more than usually taken as a vitamin supplement. In less than two months, I had to discontinue the wheat germ because severe gastrointestinal symptoms appeared. Again I was completely mystified at the turn of events because I did not find out about enzyme inhibitors until years later. Perhaps you would not feel the bad effects if you confined the dosage to one or two tablespoons.

STARCH BLOCKERS AND ENZYME DEPLETION

The latest rage amongst the diet-crazed American public is perhaps the most dangerous since the highly touted high-protein diets and appetite suppressive drugs—starch blockers. Starch blockers are special enzyme inhibitors that prevent the body's assimilation of starches. The advertisers claim that the dieter can eat strawberry shortcake and still lose weight. But what are the effects of such an apparent miraculous weight loss plan?

We can draw some conclusions from the results of a few studies in which growing rats and chickens were fed trypsin (protein) inhibitors with their food. The results included marked enlargement of the pancreas and greatly increased enzyme secretion by the pancreas, with the enzyme wastage due to excretion with the feces; weakness and failure to grow; and poor health overall. These studies are discussed more fully later in this chapter.

When protein is eaten with protein inhibitors, the pancreas secretes more enzymes than it would produce if the inhibitors were not consumed. There is no reason to disbelieve that when starch is eaten with starch inhibitors, the pancreas would produce more enzymes than when starch is consumed alone. The ingestion of any type of inhibitor also causes a great quantity of enzymes to be lost by excretion. Such heavy withdrawals from the enzyme bank account constitute a health hazard. As mentioned earlier, it has been demonstrated that when all of the pancreatic enzymes are drained out of the body and wasted, the experimental subjects died within a week. In the case of starch blockers, the effects would be slower, but would still considerably shorten life.

Preventing the normal functioning of the body is a deplorable way to achieve some dubious end such as weight control at any cost. There are people who control their weight by eating a big meal to enjoy the pleasure of eating, and then inducing vomiting to expel it. This state is similar to bulimia, and is very dangerous. It not only removes the unwanted calories from the body, but also wastes the enzymes that had been produced to digest the meal. It makes no difference if all of the enzymes are wasted via fistulae in research animals, or wasted by vomiting. Death is the result. In human or experimental intestinal obstruction, there is uninterrupted vomiting with consequent wastage of enzymes. If the obstruction is not corrected, death results within a week.

Only time will prove the deleterious effects of the starch blockers. Unfortunately, innocent victims may sacrifice sizable quantities of their precious enzymes to this dubious approach to weight loss before the truth is known.

GERMINATED NUTS AND GRAINS

In germinated tree nuts and cereal grains we can find all of the protein, carbohydrate, fat, and calories we will ever need. The world is looking for someone to put these items on the market in a palatable form, untouched by heat and free from enzyme inhibitors. I have ideas how to go about it but am not young enough to finish the job. When I started with the food-enzyme problem in 1932, I had a vague idea it could be solved in a year or two. The world desperately needs high-grade protein and fat, and tree nuts have them. But do not try subtracting these materials from their enzymes or you will end up with yet more nutritionally deficient food.

It would be a great boon to our health if germinated cereal grains were readily available on the market in raw, palatable form. As a matter of fact, germinated cereals have been made available but need to be made more palatable to be eaten raw. Even if these foods required refrigeration to maintain high quality, a big market of food-enzyme-conscious consumers should develop. I will be the first customer.

Millions of acres could be planted in nut-bearing trees. The land under and between the trees would still be available for agricultural or other use. Indeed, such large-scaled production of nuts would favor minimal cost to the consumer. A steer needs more than an acre to produce a few hundred pounds of beef. But just one acre planted in nut-bearing trees would yield far more protein and fat. With increasing world population, dwindling acreage, and difficulties with beef production, the protein situation will become acute. Increasing hospital and health care will also ultimately reach an acute stage. Complete enzyme nutrition, which the germinated nuts and cereals provide, can put a damper on the basic, if unrecognized, cause of many diseases, and solve food shortages at the same time.

I have consolidated information on enzyme inhibitors in foods in Table 7.1. It lists the material tested, the name of the enzyme inhibited, the scientists that did the research, the place where it was done, and the year the report was published.

Table 7.1

ENZYME INHIBITORS IN FOODS

Material	Enzyme Inhibited	Authority	Year	University or Institution
Wheat, rye, corn	Amylase	Kneen et al.	1946	Nebraska
Sweet potato	Trypsin	Sohonie et al.	1956	Bombay Inst. Science
Seeds and beans	Trypsin	Laskowski et al.	1954	Marquette
Soybean	Trypsin	Lyman	1957	California
Field bean	Trypsin	Banerji et al.	1969	Bombay Inst. Science
Lima bean, egg white	Trypsin	Lyman et al.	1962	California
Barley	Trypsin	Mikola et al.	1969	Helsinki Lab.
Wheat	Amylase	Militzer et al.	1946	Nebraska
Potato	Invertase	Schwimmer et al.	1961	USDA
Unripe mango, banana, and papaya	Peroxidase, amylase and catalase	Matto et al.	1970	Baroda, India
Raw wheat germ	Trypsin	Creek et al.	1962	Maryland
Egg white	Chymotrypsin, amylase	Rothman et al.	1969	Harvard
Sunflower seed	Trypsin	Agren et al.	1968	Uppsala, Sweden
Rye	Protease	Polanowski	1967	Breslau, Poland
Lettuce seed	Trypsin	Shain et al.	1968	Hebrew Univ. Israel
Wheat flour	Trypsin	Learmouth et al.	1963	British Soya Prod.
Peanut	Trypsin, chymotrypsin	Hochstrasser	1969	Muenchen, Germany
Corn and oat	Trypsin	Lorenc-Kubis	1969	Wroclaw, Poland
Potato	Trypsin	Sohonie et al.	1955	Bombay Inst. Science
Potato	Chymotrypsin	DeEds et al.	1964	USDA
Soybean	Transamidinase	Borchers	1964	Nebraska
Raw wheat, rye germs	Trypsin	Hochstrasser et al.	1969	Munich, Germany
Algae, porphyra vul.	Trypsin	Ishihara et al.	1968	Nutritional Abstracts
Squid liver	Trypsin	Ishikawa	1968	Chemical Abstracts
Radish seed	Trypsin	Ogawa	1968	Kyoto, Japan
Whole wheat flour	Trypsin	Shyamala et al.	1961	California

ENZYME INHIBITORS IN EXPERIMENTAL RESEARCH

In 1968, the scientists Y. Shain and A.M. Mayer reported experiments performed at the Hebrew University in Israel in the journal *Phytochemistry*. The following tables (7.2 and 7.3) summarize their work on the germination of lettuce seeds. It can be seen in Table 7.2 that as the enzyme trypsin is gradually released from the grip of enzyme inhibitors as germination proceeds, enzyme activity increases greatly. Trypsin is a proteolytic enzyme secreted by the pancreas. Its function is to break down protein into smaller units, such as amino acids. Table 7.3 shows that during 24 hours of germination, enzyme inhibitors were completely inactivated. This evidence can be interpreted as indicating that the great increase in enzyme activity during germination inactivates enzyme inhibitors. Other scientists have shown that adding concentrated enzymes to seeds also inactivates the inhibitors.

Table 7.2

DEVELOPMENT OF TRYPSIN ACTIVITY
WITH GERMINATION

Hours of Germination	Trypsin Activity Units
0	7.5
24	60.0
48	257.0
72	333.0

Table 7.3

DISAPPEARANCE OF TRYPSIN INHIBITORS
DURING GERMINATION

Length of Germination Hours	Inhibitor Activity Units	% Decrease From Dry Seeds
0	2.07	0
6	0.73	65
15	0.30	86
24	0.00	100

A research team of A.N. Booth and three other scientists at the California Laboratory of the US Department of Agriculture made a report in 1960 on different effects of feeding rats raw and cooked soybeans. One group of rats was fed raw soybeans, in which state the enzymes were held helpless by the accompanying enzyme inhibitors. The other group of rats ate cooked soybeans, containing neither enzymes nor inhibitors. The results are tabulated in Table 7.4. The inhibitors in the raw beans prevented the young rats from growing normally and gaining weight. At the same time, the pancreas had to fight the inhibitors with an oversecretion of pancreatic enzymes, and was forced to enlarge to do this. The scientists studied the contents of the bowel and found the enzymes were being wasted by excretion into the feces and lost. They believed this was the reason for the poor health and growth of the animals. This shows that the organism cannot tolerate waste of its enzymes.

Table 7.4
EFFECT OF SOYBEAN DIETS ON
BODY AND PANCREAS WEIGHTS OF RATS

Kind of Diet	Number of Rats	Final Body Weight Grams	Pancreas Weight (% of Body Weight)
Raw	5	89.00	0.85
Cooked	5	148.40	0.50

The effect of enzyme inhibitors on overall health, body weight, and pancreas weight has been tested on chickens, as well as rats. In 1948, a group working at the University of California (including S. Lepkovsky) used chickens. Table 7.5 shows the results of their work. On a diet of raw soybeans containing the enzyme inhibitors, the birds failed to grow and gain body weight. But this stunted growth did not apply to their pancreas glands which became more than twice as

Table 7.5
EFFECT OF SOYBEAN DIETS ON WEIGHT AND
ENZYME CONTENT OF PANCREAS OF CHICKS

Kind of Diet	Number of Chicks	Days on Diet	Body Weight Grams	Pancreas Weight Grams	Pancreas (% of Body Weight)	Protease Activity Units
Raw	19	20	127	1.21	0.96	0.38
Cooked	19	20	207	0.92	0.44	0.23

heavy as the group of birds eating cooked soybean in which the enzyme inhibitors are destroyed. The table shows a marked increase in enzyme output on the inhibitor diet, denoting a waste of precious enzymes. The enzyme potential of the organism could not stand this loss and the health and growth of the birds suffered as a result. Rats and chickens eating enzyme inhibitors in raw soybeans were sick animals.

The evidence developed by these inhibitor experiments duplicates and confirms what is recorded in other pages of this volume about the dire consequences of experimental removal of pancreatic juice enzymes from the intestinal tract.

8

Enzymes to the Rescue: The Mystique of Fasting

Some people actually fear they may die if they miss a few meals. How about not eating for a whole year? Some Oriental individuals possess remarkable control over their bodies in a manner we do not understand. The British scientist James Knight in the treatise "Suspended Animation and Kindred Subjects," speaks of the stupor trance practiced in the East. The subject goes into a deep sleep that may last for days, weeks, months, or even a year. During the period of quiescence, the pulse becomes impalpable and the respiration imperceptible. Following a well-ordered formula after coming out of the trance, the individual finally returns to normal daily activities without noticeable impairments. These trances and other such mystical feats are not understood by western science. My purpose in citing such facts is to stimulate experiments which may eventually open new avenues and explain the phenomena in terms of physical science. The paper describing these episodes was published in the *Proceedings of the Royal Philosophical Society*, Glasgow.

Mahatma Gandhi was a master strategist in the art of fasting. His fasts united the Indian populace and frightened the Imperial British forces because of the common belief that anyone who misses a few meals is headed for disaster. In fasting, Gandhi was willing to martyr himself for the cause of a unified, independent India. It is also possible that Gandhi used fasting as a way of repudiating his former, conventional lifestyle. Every time this beloved leader went on one of his fasts, the press of the day carried screaming headlines warning of his imminent demise.

Let us consider this for a moment. I believe that Gandhi unwittingly practiced a regimen of therapeutic fasting. The warm Indian climate prevented his body temperature from plummeting to a dangerous level. A reduction in physical activity also conserved enough energy to sustain him throughout his prolonged fasts. Despite symptoms of illness, Gandhi emerged from each fast to resume his role in the political struggle. It took an assassin's bullet to put an end to the life of this unusual, outwardly frail man.

From what has been said here let no one jump to the conclusion that he may start a fast as a mere lark. It should not be undertaken by the uninitiated. A short fast offers little hope of achieving substantial results, and an extended fast should only be considered if an experienced doctor is willing to assume responsibility. An extended fast may be accompanied by a more or less violent upheaval or "healing crisis." These developments must be evaluated by the doctor with care. If the vital signs, as indicated by the physical examination and supplemented by laboratory findings, are not unfavorable, there may be much to gain by continuing the fast and weathering the reactions. The old dictum about fasting until the tongue is clean has a ring of truth. But if the vitality of the organism is insufficient to sustain the changes going on during a fast, it must be terminated. In this case it should never have been started. An experienced doctor can decide this at the beginning. The uninitiated fast at their own peril.

THERAPEUTIC FASTING

Fasting has been popular among certain groups as a method of treatment for ailments since the nineteenth century. As a therapeutic measure, it commands a degree of justification. During a fast the stress on the organism for the digestion and assimilation of food and elimination of its waste is drastically reduced. The manufacture of digestive enzymes is cut down to a trickle, so the body has a better chance to supply what is needed to overhaul what is often a neglected and run-down piece of machinery. It has been estimated that 50 percent of the daily production of protein in the living organism goes for enzymes, a major share of which is for digestive enzymes. During a fast the need for digestive enzymes is eliminated. Released from the burden of some heavy chores, the enzyme potential helps to remodel the body at an accelerated pace.

In the 1920s I was on the staff of a sanitarium, and I saw about 50 instances of therapeutic fasting while I was there. The *modus operandi* in the fasting "cure" was to abstain from food for periods varying from a week up to a month. During the routine of a fast all food was prohibited and the practice was to drink a glass of water with 2 tea-spoons of orange juice in it at each mealtime. The craving for food usually vanished after 2 or 3 days. Water was taken between mealtimes and daily enemas were given at the start. During a prolonged fast, physical activity was cut down. The appearance of gastrointestinal disturbances or skin eruptions or boils within several weeks was welcomed and taken as an indication that the "healing crisis" had arrived. After several days of fasting, the tongue often gets heavily coated and may remain that way for many days.

Traditionally, in therapeutic fasting, unlike fasting to correct obesity, one of the objects is to lose as little weight as possible. A fast is taboo if the weight is on the low side. Fasting is avoided in the cold months to prevent dissipating the energy needed to maintain body temperature. Although many persons have undertaken a fast on their own initiative, it is wise to have at least a rudimentary physical examination to determine if there are any contraindications. During the duration of a fast, periodic check-ups are imperative.

I have a record on file of a visit by a man on January 28, 1925. He came to me on the twenty-second day of a fast and was becoming weak. He undertook the fast in winter and on his own volition. He stated his original weight as 143 pounds. His record shows the following:

Weight: 119½ pounds
Pulse: 40
Systolic blood pressure: 84 (He stated it was 118 originally.)
Oral temperature: 93.3° F at 2:00 pm
Tongue fairly clean and pink
Breath not offensive
Heart sounds weakened but normal

The patient had taken nothing but water for 22 days, and during that period he had used periodic enemas. When he tried to return to food, his stomach would not retain it, and vomiting resulted. Because of the gravity of the situation it was obvious that this man should be under constant supervision. He was taken in at the sanitarium and started on hourly feedings of a spoonful of fresh fruit juice, and later, milk. In a few days he could return to normal food and retain it. Once the danger had been weathered, the patient claimed that his original complaint, upper respiratory "catarrh," had been improved by the fast. This man undertook this fast for therapeutic reasons, not for reducing. He claimed improvement in symptoms. I don't believe it harmed his body. Persons undertaking a fast should be under professional guidance so the body functions can be monitored.

Not much impression can be made on a chronic ailment in a few days. It may require several weeks of fasting. In many cases when the "crisis" or change-over period arrives, various symptoms appear. These may take the form of skin eruptions and gastrointestinal disturbances manifested by foul breath, coated tongue, flatulence, or nausea. During my tenure on the staff of the sanitarium, less than half of the therapeutic fasters experienced these crises (which were considered beneficial). People felt cheated if they did not get theirs. The M.D. in charge of the sanitarium had studied in European spas, bringing the crisis philosophy home with him.

By and large, the regular medical profession has never been greatly enthused about therapeutic fasting. It may sound strange to the ears of orthodox medicine, but I have seen results from fasting in chronic disease patients. In the healing crisis, the system purges itself of infiltrations that are at the root of some systemic ailments. Perhaps when the organism is relieved of its usual chores for an extended period, it accumulates enough enzyme power to autolyze (dissolve) some pathological conditions by virtue of being able to concentrate more intense enzyme activity on them.

Therapeutic fasting enjoyed a degree of vogue in a former generation, if the titles of books in that era are any indication. Upton Sinclair, the famous novelist, wrote one in 1911 entitled, *The Fasting Cure*. Another, *The True Science of Living, The New Gospel of Health, The Story of an Evolution of Natural Law and the Cure of Disease, For Physicians and Laymen, How the Sick Get Well, How the Well Get Sick,* was written by Reverend George Edward Hooker Dewey in 1908. *Fasting for Health and Life,* by Dr. Josiah Oldfield (1924), and *Fasting for the Cure of Disease,* by Dr. Linda B. Hazzard (1908), are other examples that suggest that the expectation from fasting was to lose much more than just pounds. These fasters wanted to get rid of their disease troubles.

Some years ago, I read a magazine piece entitled "Autolyze Your Tumors." The author, a doctor, argued that enzyme activity of the body, under certain conditions, could digest and dissolve tumors. With this I have had no experience. H.C. Bradley, University of Wisconsin (1922), gives these examples of physiological autolysis, which is nothing more than enzyme action within the tissues:

- Atrophy of mammary gland after lactation.
- Atrophy of uterus after parturition.
- Atrophy from immobilization.
- Atrophy of tadpole's tail during metamorphosis.

If my memory serves, there are instances in medical reports where kidney stones have been dissolved during the course of pregnancy and other specific physiological states. Radiographs show that the excessive callous formation at the site of fractures is dissolved in due course. Callous formation is caused by calcium which deposits around a fracture site to "cement" the parts together. After the fracture is healed, the extra calcium is reabsorbed. These restorative processes are instances of physiological autolysis and can take place only through the agency of enzyme action and when the organism is in a particular physiological state. It is not unreasonable to suggest that under the conditions existing at a certain stage of a prolonged fast, such a state exists. It is the most logical explanation for some of the modest results which I have observed from fasting in arthritis and chronic disease in patients.

FASTING TO LOSE WEIGHT

About 30 years ago physicians became interested in fasting for obesity in cases that resisted other methods of treatment. Persons with weights of approximately 500 pounds cannot depend on exercise to burn fat; strenuous physical activity is out of the quesiton. So the medical literature started to pick up a bit on fasting. In one series of cases the fasting was undertaken in a facility connected with the University of California.

In 1964 a report was made on results obtained by Drs. Drenick, Swendseid, Blahd, and Tuttle in the *Journal of the American Medical Association*. They studied 11 patients ranging in weight from 236 to 550 pounds. They fasted for periods varying from 12 to 117 days at the University of California facility. Weight losses averaged slightly less than 1 pound per day. The greatest weight loss in a single period of fasting was 116 pounds in 117 days of fasting. The authors claim 117 days is a record for a single fast. This occurred in a woman 39 years of age, who originally weighed 315 pounds. Many of the persons in the group had hypertension or arteriosclerotic heart disease. The blood pressure returned to normal after fasting. During the period of the fast only water and vitamins were consumed.

FASTING AND ARTHRITIS

There are indications fasting has a way of relieving the organism of some of the deposits identified with atherosclerosis and arthritis.

In most instances an elevated blood pressure is reduced. Bronchial symptoms may recede. Likewise some gastrointestinal troubles may relax their grip, resulting in better digestion and more normal evacuation of the bowels. "Allergic" congestion and fullness of the nasopharyngeal region usually improve. A successful fast may reward the participant with definite improvement in arthritis. One cannot stay on a fast long enough to effect a "cure" in deforming arthritis.

ENZYMES AND ARTHRITIS

Dr. Arnold Renshaw of Manchester, England, has dealt with many cases through the enzyme approach. His report in the *Annals of Rheumatic Disease* (1947) has remained buried and hidden far too long. Dr. Renshaw noted that "Many theories have been advanced from time to time to explain the etiology of rheumatic diseases." He added that in this connection the functions of the small intestine have received little notice and less research. "As a result of numerous postmortem examinations, sometimes as many as 4 or 6 a day, for many years, the frequency with which atrophy of the small intestine occurred and the variations in the appearance of this organ when it was systematically opened and examined throughout its entire length, impressed itself upon the writer. The conclusion was reached that rheumatoid arthritis might be a deficiency disease arising from an inability to deal adequately with protein digestion and metabolism. It is to be noted that the area of the small intestine, excluding folds and villi, is at least 9 or 10 times that of the stomach, and Martin and Banks of McGill University (1940) showed that the weight of the dried intestinal mucosa is from 3 to 5 times that of the dried pancreas."

Dr. Renshaw decided to test his theory that an enzyme shortage is behind arthritis. A firm of enzyme specialists produced a dried enzyme extract of the intestinal mucosa. Persons with rheumatic ailments swallowed the enzyme in capsule form after meals. As many as 7 capsules were taken each day. Treatment was carried out at a clinic at Ancoats Hospital, Manchester, and in private practice. Among more than 700 private patients treated with the enzyme over a period of 7 years, good results were obtained in rheumatoid arthritis, osteoarthritis, fibrositis (an inflammation of connective tissue). Some intractable cases of ankylosing spondylitis (an inflammation of the vertebrae that causes stiffening) and Still's disease (which affects youngsters, involving many joints and sometimes retarding development) have also responded to this therapy. In a series of 556 cases of various types, 283 were found to be much improved, and a further 219 were improved to a less marked extent. Of 292 cases of rheumatoid arthritis, 264 showed improvement of various degrees. Improvement was also noted in other forms of rheumatism. Children with Still's disease responded very well in a few cases treated, and relief of pain was frequently reported by patients with osteoarthritis.

It was further pointed out that for the first two or three months there may be no noticeable improvement; in fact the pain may become slightly worse. The longer the duration of the disease, the longer the lag before improvement is observed. Persons with arthritis of more than 5 years duration may require 6 to 12 months of treatment with the enzyme capsules before improvement in the rheumatic condition becomes obvious. Nevertheless if treatment is persistently maintained, in due course, this class of case will show definite response. In certain cases Dr. Renshaw observed that it required 18 months to 2 years for the sedimentation rate to approach normal.

My own experience with a different type of enzyme capsule has been similar to Dr. Renshaw's with respect to the time element involved to show some improvement in the worst cases of long-standing osteoarthritis and rheumatoid arthritis. It is the same story with raw diets in these advanced conditions. It is a slow process. But if a victim of these incapacitating maladies decides there may be another 5 to 10 years of life left, isn't it worth proceeding along such slow but constructive lines? Massive dosage, i.e., more frequent ingestion of capsules each day, may speed up the process. But massive enzyme therapy requires observation under a doctor with blood tests to determine how many capsules can be tolerated each day. Each case is different. However, there are no side effects such as occur with the use of cortisone. One fault with enzyme treatment of arthritis is finding a doctor with the patience to carry it out long enough to show some results!

CANCER AND ENZYMES

Like arthritis, cancer is a complex problem that requires medical observation if enzyme therapy is to be employed.

Because of the unrelenting mortality rate from cancer and its close identification with changes in enzyme chemistry, cancer stands out as the Number One candidate for massive enzyme therapy. There is abundant laboratory proof of profoundly disturbed enzyme chemistry in cancer. Viewed through the eyes of Enzyme Nutrition and the

Food Enzyme Concept, the choice of massive enzyme therapy as the indicated and preferred approach to the cancer problem is clear. Examinations of cancer tissue have shown that while the level of many enzymes is below normal, some enzymes have a level higher than normal. These tests have been done for a long time on human material by many investigators and involved a variety of enzymes. More recently the tests were performed on animal cancer, but not on the spontaneous variety. It is easy for researchers to develop animal cancer in the laboratory, but difficult to look for and find the spontaneous variety.

In searching to explain the high level of these "rescue" enzymes we have to consider the possibility they represent the response of the organism to drastic methods of therapy such as surgery, radiation, and chemotherapy.

I have been interested in the cancer problem for many years, but have not been satisfied with the character of cancer research on laboratory animals. The aim of most of this research is not so much to identify the basic cause of cancer, but to discover chemical compounds which hold cancer in check temporarily, but cannot prevent it from slowly continuing its killing course. But a somewhat different approach is suggested by Dr. Knox of Harvard Medical School with his book *Enzyme Patterns in Fetal, Adult and Neoplastic Rat Tissue.* Knox writes: "It will come as a surprise to scientists in other fields, and even to some biologists that we do not yet know the rudimentary composition of different living tissues." Dr. Knox stresses that science should develop enzyme physiology and enzyme anatomy, which is precisely what I have been involved in these many years. His book lists the concentration of 161 enzymes in 17 rat tissues. (The term "neoplastic" referred to in the book title means "cancerous.") Dr. Knox's work was meant to establish normal enzyme values in rat tissues which could then be compared with the enzyme values in rat cancer. One theory behind such investigations is that if one or more enzymes are consistently found in subnormal amount, these enzymes can then be administered to human cancer patients. Cancer is induced in laboratory rats that are then used to test cancer remedies that have shown promise in controlling cancer. The problem with the procedures is that cancer in rats is not the same as cancer in humans.

Problems With Enzyme Testing in Cancer Research

Rat cancer is developed by such drastic methods as injecting cancer cells into the blood of rats or grafting cancer tissue on their bodies.

The resulting cancer is a far cry from cancer in humans, which arises spontaneously. If a remedy has shown good results in human cancer and is then used on artificial rat cancer and fails to reproduce the same results, it proves nothing because the two kinds of cancer are as dissimilar—as far apart—as the positive and negative poles of a magnet.

This approach to the problem is not sound because the test animals are not representative of human cancer. If a certain enzyme in a given cancer tissue gave a low test reading in the animals with artificial cancer, this may be completely misleading because the same enzyme in the corresponding human tissue afflicted with spontaneous cancer may test normal. To have any legitimacy and real meaning, this approach to cancer must utilize animals with spontaneous cancer. But to find such animal subjects is time-consuming and impractical. And objections would be raised if samples of cancer tissue in living persons were cut out for testing, particularly if the malignancy involved an internal organ. Furthermore, post-mortem tests on human spontaneous cancer sometimes disclose high values for some enzymes in certain tissues. These are "rescue" enzymes. This is my own term, based on my theory that when cancer is treated by x-ray or surgery, the organism reacts and sends enzymes to repair the secondary tissue damage caused by this type of therapy. This is the only logical explanation I could find for elevated enzyme values at a cancer site.

One after another the chemicals making up the formulas of commonly advertised remedies are being accused of causing cancer as a result of testing on laboratoy rats and mice. Other chemical compounds used around the home have been tested and found to be carcinogenic (cancer-causing) and banned from the market. Cancer researchers feel they are serving society and doing their duty by this sort of detective work. But from what you have learned by studying this book, you know they are merely pointing at stimulating factors of cancer, and not the one basic cause. If the body chemistry is not afflicted by the basic cause, the hundreds of stimulating causes will be ineffective in causing cancer.

An African watering hole supplies drinking water to hundreds of animals, and although it is dirty and carries dozens of questionable and possibly carcinogenic chemicals, none of them become ill from it. The animals are protected by their superb body chemistry and maintained by a raw diet from which no enzyme nutrients have been removed. What do you suppose would happen to a hundred people if they habitually drank from such a water hole? The fear of bacterial attack is a deterring factor. What is the reason for the immunity of wild animals against disease under these conditions? Wild animals of the deep jungle, far removed from human machinations, are singularly free from all human-type degenerative, intractable ailments. All of these creatures get everything in the food that grew in it, including the food enzymes. On the other hand, humans started to receive fewer food enzymes when they learned to cook and completed the trend to an enzymeless diet with the advent of the modern automatic kitchen and food factory. From what you have learned about the Food Enzyme Concept, you can say that if cancer researchers tested some carcinogens on wild rats, eating their natural raw diet, the rats would not become cancer victims. It is only when rats are born and raised on the factory, enzymeless chow diet (no raw food at all), that they become targets for cancer. Let us carry this a step farther. Instead of wild rats, take ordinary laboratory rats and feed them a raw diet, plus carcinogens, and see what happens. Carry it still farther, use a factory diet and carcinogens on laboratory rats, plus enzyme supplements, the diet and supplements to be divided into many feedings throughout the day.

My handling of the cancer phenomenon is totally different from the direct attack. The principles of Enzyme Nutrition and the Food Enzyme Concept disallow direct, specific treatment of cancer. The proper course is to make it unnecessary for the digestive system to produce so many digestive enzymes so the enzyme potential will have the capacity to make and channel more metabolic enzymes to the site of malignancy and normalize its enzyme chemistry. The result from this course of action depends to some extent on the cancer victim's understanding of the philosophy of Enzyme Nutrition and his enthusiasm in carrying it out. Even in terminal cancer patients whose tissues have been abused and damaged, the desire to forge ahead can make the difference between success and failure.

Earlier in this volume I explained that it is necessary to drastically tame down overly rich digestive enzyme secretions so that metabolic enzyme potency can be increased to an effective level. A complete fast reduces digestive enzyme secretion to a trickle in several days. This would enable the enzyme potential to effectively remodel any area involved in defective metabolism. But the victims of terminal cancer are poor candidates for a fast long enough to be effective.

Enzyme Therapy for Cancer

Let us briefly summarize what has been presented to this point. To avoid or deal with disease, the body must be continually reinforced with good protein, vitamins, and minerals. But to eat these materials in a proper diet is not enough. It requires expert mechanics to build these materials into blood, nerves, organs, and tissues. That means enzyme power—metabolic enzymes. Only these enzymes know how to structure proteins, vitamins, and minerals into the tissues of your body. If you must allot much of your enzyme power for digestion, and less for running your body, you are inviting diseases. The situation is something like trying to stretch a pint of paint to paint a house. But if outside enzymes help with digestion, you will have plenty of enzyme power to run the body properly, promote feelings of well-being, and prevent countless ailments.

Because there is no proof that spontaneous human cancer and experimental laboratory cancer are identical, there is no reason why massive enzyme therapy cannot be used directly in human cancer, instead of employing it first on animals. Being nontoxic, enzymes are in a different class than the ordinary toxic chemotherapy compounds. If massive enzyme therapy were used on laboratory cancer, there is a strong possibility a negative result would lead to a false interpretation that massive enzyme therapy is without value in spontaneous human cancer. If animals must be used, they should be of a strain developing spontaneous cancer.

I offer a program involving a special diet and massive enzyme supplements. This could be properly carried out only in a hospital where the vital signs of the patient are periodically monitored and recorded. Such a regimen might involve frequent small meals and oral administration of enzymes every half hour. Therefore the necessity for careful supervision is obvious, especially in terminal cancer cases. The cost of this program of special hospital care can be expected to be high. It would be unreasonable to expect cancer patients to pay for this intensive course of Enzyme Nutrition until it has been proven on a large scale. Most of them have already exhausted their resources. But I believe that if money were available to pay for this hospital program, it would make far more than a ripple in cancer management. It would make headlines from coast to coast. No buildings necessary. No expensive laboratories to build. All of the money would be spent for hospital expenses catering to cancer victims.

BEATING ALLERGIES

Let's talk about allergies involving certain raw foods using strawberries as an example. Do you break out from eating strawberries? Keep eating them! But eat only one a day. Yes, only one strawberry a day.

If you still itch or break out, eat only a piece each day. When your system can tolerate this reaction, go back up to one berry a day. Then increase to one berry twice each day. Then one 3 times each day, 2 hours after meals. Some persons can jump from here to a few berries 3 times a day and then increase to a small dish 3 times a day without a reaction. Others cannot get away with it yet. They may have to settle for one berry every 2 hours, 8 times a day and try building up later. This takes time. It may require weeks or months to restore a tolerance for the food. The aim is to work up a tolerance so a dishful of the food can be taken at one time without reaction. If any reactions occur, it is an indication that smaller and more frequent feedings are in order. The same routine is applicable to any raw food to which one is allergic. All of this trouble would hardly be worthwhile just to be able to eat a single food. But something far more important is at stake. Being "allergic" to a raw food may be nature's way of telling us that the food's enzymes are incompatible with some unwholesome bodily condition, and are on the warpath to overpower it!

There is nothing new about this system of increasing tolerances. I was familiar with it a few years before the term allergy was coined (about 1924), as a result of a very unpleasant experience I had at the tender age of twelve. I was afflicted with what is now called allergic rhinitis (congestive). I was a "mouth breather" because of completely clogged up nasal passages. On the advice of the family doctor, my folks consulted a specialist who taught at Rush Medical College. He advised surgery. We assumed that meant cure. After the turbinate cartilage was surgically removed, I returned to his clinic once a week for several months. One of the doctors would pick up an applicator tipped with cotton and dip it into a mysterious solution (adrenalin?) and probe the nostrils several times. After several months of this, I finally asked how long it would take for a cure. I still remember being shocked when the doctor told me there was no cure for the condition.

In retrospect, I now believe this unhappy turbinectomy was the best thing that could have happened to me. It taught me to be on guard and suspicious, especially in matters of health. When a health problem comes up, I always look for a non-surgical approach. Incidentally, turbinectomy was given up as a bad deal years ago when the allergy concept arrived—but not before millions had the useless operation. One of the reports that helped to usher out the era of promiscuous turbinectomies is found in the *Journal of the American Medical Association* in 1925. Here is what Drs. Piness and Miller wrote about some patients under the title "Allergy: A Nonsurgical Disease of the Nose and Throat": "In a group of 834 allergic patients there were 704 operative procedures on the nose and throat without relief, there having been no removal of the offending allergen. Since there is an increasing risk of untoward operative sequelae with so large a number of operations, we urge that allergic manifestations be classified as nonoperative conditions of the respiratory tract. Allergy of the respiratory membranes is a clinical entity."

Some years after having the turbinectomy I found out how to beat allergic rhinitis by using measures similar to those mentioned above. The nasal membranes shrunk to the point where normal breathing was possible.

Let's return to allergic reactions manifested by itching, burning, or an eruption of the skin. One way of looking at these is that they are outward manifestations of the body's displeasure in having to deal with a food not agreeable to it. Look at it another way. How do we know that the itching, burning, and eruption are not caused by the escape of some unwholesome material nature is attempting to purge by throwing it out? Is it not possible that strawberries (for example) possess some remedial agent, such as enzymes, which may work on various types of noxious substrates infiltrating the body? Enzymes are very active agents. In the laboratory a particular enzyme must have its own specific substrate. A starch enzyme will not work on protein. If a raw-food enzyme finds its substrate in the body it will work on it. If that substrate is a pernicious foreign material, the product of the enzyme reaction may be something the body cannot tolerate. In that case the body would try getting rid of it by throwing it out through the skin. This effort may show up as the symptoms of allergy.

Scavenger Enzymes

There are various types of metabolic enzymes, including scavenger enzymes. In order to build a product a factory needs materials of various kinds, such as steel, brass, plastics, and so on. But these would not be able to realize final form without the workers. And foremen are also needed to direct the workers. In the living body, protein, fat, carbohydrate, vitamins, and minerals are the materials to work with. The enzymes are the workers, and the hormones are foremen. In a factory, waste material is part of the normal operation. A scavenger crew is kept busy removing it. In the living body the scavenging is done by special enzymes, scavenger enzymes, if you will. These special enzyme deputies cruise about in the blood looking for dead, inert, and offensive material, in a fashion comparable to the vultures circulating around in a tropical sky with the task of keeping the landscape wholesome. Some of our scavenger enzymes are present in white blood cells. The functions of these scavengers include the attempt to prevent the arteries from clogging up and the joints from being crammed with arthritic deposits. If scavenger enzymes find the right substrate they latch on and reduce it to a form the blood can dispose of. If the scavenger enzymes cannot handle the load, nature may throw some of the unwanted material out through the skin, or perhaps through the membranes of the nose and throat, producing the familiar postnasal drip. Not nice, but isn't it better than allowing the "factory waste" to pile up in the arteries, joints, or tissues and create diseases? Here is where TV nostrums step in, claiming to shrink membranes in the nose. These inefficacious remedies could cause the condition to be chased into the middle ear via the eustachian tube, initiating deafness later. It may require a bundle of money for research to prove or disprove this thesis, but, unfortunately that money is not forthcoming.

In the meantime, why not experiment with the offending raw fruits or vegetables in tolerable amounts. It is best to reduce the food to a juice if possible. Find out by personal experiment if the enzymes in the food cannot exhaust the allergic tendencies of the body. For instance, if you cannot tolerate fresh raw orange juice, start taking it in amounts of a half teaspoon, say 3 times a day. As tolerance increases, work up to every 2 hours, 8 times a day. Gradually increase the dose to a tablespoonful, then a quarter glass, and finally a full glass 3 times a day. One should understand that real effort and patience applied to this routine may be rewarded with some very pleasant changes in the body. It goes without saying that only raw, ripe fruit should be used. Try to comprehend that when the allergy goes, something much more serious in the body may likewise be set right. If an allergy is conquered in this fashion, there is reason to expect improvement in some symptom or bodily condition that may be far removed from the site of the allergic symptoms. For instance, when there are no more allergic reactions to a particular raw food, there may also be improvement in the lungs, stomach, or nose and throat. Time will tell. I have seen persons permanently relieved of allergic symptoms from certain raw foods. Certain symptoms can return if one goes back to an offensive nutritionally unbalanced diet. Call it a cure or whatever you like. Is this long-distance doctoring? It is sometimes difficult to get the whole story about the body even after going through the rigamarole of a good hospital, and any kind of absentee doctoring can be disappointing, even the doctor columns of newspapers. But how would the average reader go about testing an idea like this? If a cooperating doctor can be found to watch your case, so much the better.

Research on Enzymes for Allergies

Regarding the influence of administration of enzymes by physicians in treatment of ailments, many of which were presumed to have an allergic basis, the medical literature has a number of contributions. In other reports where enzymes were employed the object of the treatment was to supplement a deficient secretion of digestive enzymes. Dr. A.W. Oelgoetz wrote a report entitled, "The Treatment of Food Allergy," published in the *Medical Record* in 1936. He advised use of whole pancreas powder (not pancreatin) in ailments showing positve reaction to a particular blood test. According to his theory, food allergy results when the protease, amylase, and lipase in the blood fall below a certain level, allowing unhydrolyzed food substances to accumulate in the blood. When a patient's blood did not measure up to the standard, treatment by enzymes was indicated. Swallowing the pancreas enzymes restored the proper blood enzyme level, the undigested food particles were eliminated, and the food allergy was overcome.

The theoretical basis of Dr. Oelgoetz's concept was rejected by H.C. Bradley (1936) of the University of Wisconsin, among others. In his zeal to explain the results obtained by the treatment, Dr. Oelgoetz employed a laboratory test which Bradley and the others do not accept. But that is no cause, as pointed out by Professor Bradley, for invalidating the results obtained by the treatment. In considering these results some consideration should be given to his use of whole, dried, powdered pancreas, instead of the commonly employed pancreatin. Dr. Oelgoetz had excellent results from use of enzymes by mouth where the blood test indicated need for enzymes. He recorded the following conditions responding where the test was positive:

- Chronic angioneurotic edema.
- Allergic eczema.
- Pancreatic indigestion.
- Allergic headache.
- Allergic vomiting.
- Chronic urticaria (hives).
- Allergic edema.
- Allergic colitis.
- Pancreatic achylia.

In 1935, Oelgoetz reported his experience in treating 100 cases of allergy. He found that dosages from 75 to 90 grams of enzymes daily were required to achieve success. In 1937, O. Zajicek reported in a foreign medical journal under the title, "Therapy of Migraine in Women and of Other Allergic Disease With Oxidase." W.D. Sansum, Potter Metabolic Clinic, Santa Barbara, California, is another investigator who appears to have had considerable experience in treating allergy-based ailments with large doses of enzymes. His 1932 report, "The Treatment of Indigestion, Underweight and Allergy with the Old and New Forms of Digestive Agents," gives the degrees of response listed below in Table 8.1. Dr. Sansum employed fungal amylase, pepsin, and pancreatic enzymes.

Table 8.1
DIET-RELATED HEALTH IMPROVEMENT

Number of Cases	% Improved
34 Bronchial Asthma	88
12 Food Asthma	92
42 Food Eczema	83
19 Hay Fever	80
11 Loose Bowels	100
54 Normal Weight	Remained Constant
29 Overweight	93
197 Underweight	91
29 Urticaria or Hives	86

Dr. Sansum stressed that use of large doses of enzymes requires professional supervision. He also suggested that allergy appeared to be due, in part at least, to absorption of incompletely digested protein molecules.

It is interesting to note in the report by Dr. Sansum that persons of normal weight did not experience any weight change. On the other hand, those below normal weight gained. This weight gain is understandable because if there is a deficiency of digestive enzymes, the digestion and absorption of food are impaired. But to explain how overweight people could lose weight, as the above report indicates, it is necessary to assume that the swallowed enzymes prepare food in such a way that it does not over-stimulate the absorptive powers. More research is needed to determine whether this is the true explanation. For the time being we can dismiss the seeming paradox with the observation that blowing on the hands can warm them in winter and cool them in summer, all with the same breath.

9

Taking Lipase to Heart

Heart disease is responsible for more deaths in America than any other single problem. As a result, millions of dollars in research monies and hundreds of laboratory studies have been performed to find the cause and possible solutions to the problem. To date, however, no permanent answers have been found. Probably the closest doctors have come to reducing the incidence of heart disease is in having patients reduce the amounts of fats and cholesterol they eat. But is this the answer? Or is the lack of enzymes in these cooked fatty foods, which results in incomplete digestion and artery accumulation, at fault?

In this chapter I will discuss the role of the fat-splitting enzyme, lipase, in controlling and possibly reversing cardiovascular disease caused by the accumulation of excessive fats and cholesterol in the blood and arteries.

LIPASE AND THE CONTROL
OF CARDIOVASCULAR DISEASE

Cholesterol is a substance akin to fat and is the principal agent that clogs arteries. This clogged condition is known as atherosclerosis or arteriosclerosis. "Cardiovascular disease" is a general term referring to ailments of the heart and blood vessels.

Some authorities believe, as do I, that in certain cardiovascular diseases, fatty metabolism is impaired, even reaching back to faulty fat digestion in the digestive tract. Poor enzyme activity, especially lipase activity, is clearly a factor in these diseases. It meets the requirements of the code of physiology to have different enzymes work on

145

the same substrate, as food journeys along the digestive tract. For instance, starch is worked on by salivary amylase in the stomach, by pancreatic juice amylase in the upper intestine, and by intestinal amylase further down. It has been discovered that some proteases may produce end products that are structurally different from the end products produced by other proteases. A diversity of enzymes from different sources may be good for the living organism. Trypsin has trouble with native (raw, unheated) protein, but has no difficulty with it after pepsin works on it. In a somewhat similar fashion, it is possible that when lipase from an outside source works on fat in the food-enzyme stomach, it induces certain changes that enable pancreatic lipase to create a better finished product than when it must do the entire job alone. During the time starch is being acted upon by salivary amylase in the cardiac and fundic portions of the stomach, fat and protein are also being predigested in the food-enzyme stomach by outside protease and lipase, and thus prepared for continued digestion by pancreatic lipase and trypsin.

Before the days of pasteurization, a man might have carried a dinner pail to work containing two or more sandwiches. Each slice of bread would have been spread with a heavy layer of raw butter, with a slab of meat between the slices. Nothing I know of could prevent the lipase in that butter from having a digestive effect on the fat in the cooked meat. The lipase in the butter had a chance to melt, soak in, and predigest the fat in the meat for several hours prior to the noon meal. After the meal, there was additional time for predigestion of the meat fat by butter lipase in the food-enzyme stomach. Unpasteurized butter had far more than a little lipase. Many years ago I corresponded with a doctor who got good results in psoriasis by having patients consume several pounds of raw country butter each week. Dr. A.B. Grubb knew nothing of lipase in butter, using the method empirically. This type of lipase wizardry can have far-reaching effects, even influencing the metabolism of cholesterol. Cholesterol did not harm millions of people in former times when they lived on dairy products containing lipase. Recall that isolated Eskimos ate lots of raw meat and blubber with lipase intact, and had not a bit of atherosclerosis. Incidentally, modern butter, which lacks lipase, is now considered one of the worst offenders in cardiovascular pathology.

CHOLESTEROL AND ATHEROSCLEROSIS

In recent times a great furor has arisen about the tendency of animal fats to increase the tendency of cholesterol to settle in the arteries and cause trouble in the body. It has been found that the crystal clear "purified" vegetable oils do not raise the blood cholesterol level. There are dozens of reports in the periodic scientific literature during the last 50 years proclaiming that wherever the chemist finds fat in nature, he also finds the enzyme lipase. Lipase is present in human fat tissue and has also been found in the fat of chickens, turkeys, geese, rats, pigs, cattle, lambs, rabbits, dogs, and seals. Lipase is also found in oil-bearing seeds such as castor bean, soybean, and flax seed, in wheat and barley seeds, and in the fungus *Aspergillus flavus*. Furthermore, it is present in butter from unpasteurized milk, olives, cotton seeds, and coconuts (but not in olive oil, cottonseed oil, or coconut oil). Contrary to this seeming homogeneity in nature, modern sophisticated man seems to be a law unto himself. A European investigator reported the fat in human obesity and in fatty tumors to have less lipase than in normal fatty tissues.

In 1962, 3 British doctors decided to try to find out why cholesterol settles in and clogs arteries. Drs. C.W.M. Adams, O.B. Bayliss, and M.Z. Ibrahim tested the enzymes in normal and hardened human arteries. They found that all enzymes studied became progressively weaker in the arteries as persons became older and also as the hardening became more severe. The enzymes tested were DPN diaphorase, lactic dehydrogenase, ATP-ase, adenosine-5-monophosphatase, and cytidine triphosphatase. All of these arterial enzymes were decreased in cases of atherosclerosis. These doctors believe that a shortage of enzymes is part of a mechanism which allows cholesterol deposits to accumulate in the inner part of the arterial walls. Blood tests carried out in 1958 by L.O. Pilgeram of Stanford University demonstrated that there is a progressive decline in lipase in the blood of atherosclerosis patients with advancing middle and old age.

As if to show that humans have no monopoly on arterial hardening, in 1968 Rubinstein and his associates at Montefiore Hospital, New York, tested the blood of dogs with atherosclerosis. It is not surprising that dogs have many "human" diseases, since they are given only canned or packaged heat-treated, enzyme-free food. These doctors tested the dog blood for the metabolic enzymes dehydrogenase and reductase. They found the enzymes low to very low; worse in the advanced cases.

About 25 years ago, doctors at Michael Reese Hospital in Chicago undertook some rather exhaustive investigations on the enzyme content of the saliva, pancreatic secretion, and blood of human subjects, including the very old. They found that most of the enzymes became weaker with advancing age. The doctors, Becker, Meyer, and

Necheles, found in older persons the enzyme lipase was low, with slow fat absorption from the intestine. They speculated that in hardening of the arteries, fat may be absorbed in the unhydrolyzed state. Lipase extracted from animal pancreas was fed to both young and old subjects. Following use of the enzyme there was definite improvement in the character of fat utilization.

There is evidence throughout this manuscript that indicates that when fats, whether animal or vegetable, are eaten along with their associated enzymes, no harmful effect on the arteries or heart results. No atherosclerosis comes about. All fatty foods contain lipase in their natural state. Cooking or processing removes it. I have found there is no evidence of heart or blood vessel disease among wild animals consuming large quantities of fat. There is no evidence of these afflictions in whole nations of people eating foods containing fat when taken raw.

Millions of wild creatures eat animal fats without suffering ill effects from cholesterol. Many different civilizations throughout history used large amounts of raw milk, cream, butter, and cheese, and maintained a high standard of health, comparatively free from cardiovascular impairment due to cholesterol deposits. The reason for this immunity is suggested by the following recital of evidence, but needs to be confirmed by controlled animal research and clinical application in humans.

Whales: Big on Fats—Healthy Arteries

Dr. Maynard Murray, a research scientist, once casually mentioned to me that as a younger man he was a member of an expedition in which his duties included dissecting several hundred whales. He emphasized that he found healthy arteries in these whales, with no evidence of arteriosclerosis or cholesterol pathology. The cardiovascular system proved to be entirely normal and free from disease. This is remarkable because these whales are surrounded by 3 to 6 inches of fat and blubber under their skin, which is needed to insulate these warm-blooded mammals from the frigid water in which they live. These whales ingest large fishes, squids, and seals that offer large stores of fat. The question that must be answered is how they can do this without being punished by cholesterol deposits which their heavy use of animal fat could be expected to promote. Some whales feed on small floating or weakly swimming plant and animal organisms. In warm waters these small creatures require less fat. Whales feeding on them get less fat in the diet. Living in warm water, they do not require so much fat. But in cold, northern waters, both predator and prey need more fat, and the whale ingests large quantities of fat in everything consumed. Dr. Murray has never before published his important research although science is literally starving for such basic data. It is included as an appendix to this book.

The importance of Dr. Murray's findings becomes magnified when we realize that scientists have failed to find a single instance of heart or blood vessel disease in wild meat-eating land animals living in the deep jungle. Furthermore, as shown in Chapter 3, before the age of pasteurized milk and its products, whole nations of people lived on raw milk, butter, cream, and cheese, which contained the enzyme lipase. Many of these people reached advanced age without developing cardiovascular disease. Could it be that raw milk contains something missing in the pasteurized product, which protects the body from the ravages of cholesterol—the same cholesterol that pasteurized milk and its products are reputed to inflict upon its users?

NUTRITIONAL DANGER: FAT WITHOUT LIPASE

The easiest way to separate fat from its lipase enzymes is to destroy the lipase by cooking. I believe that this heat preparation of food is related to the bad reputation of cholesterol. The trouble starts in the human digestive tract when fat, divorced from its lipase companion, is forced to remain idle and unaltered in the stomach during the period of 2, 3, or more hours after it is swallowed. While salivary amylase and then pepsin predigest carbohydrate and protein in the stomach, lipase is absent, delaying the digestion of fat. But when fat is eaten raw, with its lipase undamaged by heat, it can be digested along with protein and carbohydrate in the upper (food-enzyme) stomach prior to the time the acidity becomes strong enough to prevent further action.

When commercial fat, deprived of its lipase companion, confronts hydrochloric acid in the human stomach, it faces a harsh experience. It may be left with a structural defect, or imprinted with some undesirable trademark that prevents it from being properly digested in the intestine. Thus it may be improperly metabolized when it reaches the body tissues later. It must be remembered that in both animals and humans, it is impossible to prevent fat plus lipase from engaging in initial digestion during the first hour in the stomach.

It has been shown in Chapter 1 that even salivary amylase, which is more effective on starch near neutral pH, digests in the cardiac and fundic portion of the stomach for a period approaching an hour. The lipase associated with fat, in common with other food enzymes, has a pH optimum farther down on the acid side of the pH scale (i.e., closer to 0), and therefore can be expected to digest fat in the upper food-enzyme stomach for a period at least as long as salivary amylase can work on starch. This happens every day in the stomachs of millions of wild animals, and before the cooking era, evolution contrived to make it a regularly scheduled event in the human stomach. And this may well be the reason that humans and animals that eat raw fat with its lipase component are immune to cardiovascular disease. In Westernized culture, however, fat digestion has been interfered with. Thus a strong reason emerges why research to explore this promising area is long overdue, and merits top priority for allocation of research funds.

LIPASE AND GOOD HEALTH IN ESKIMOS

Before the coming of the airplane, the primitive isolated Eskimo was a heavy eater of raw fat and blubber, but paradoxically, was acknowledged by medical authorities to be substantially free from heart and blood vessel disease, and most other ailments of civilization. Although the inroads of our society have now changed the lifestyle of the Eskimo, luckily there are extensive scientific records attesting to the facts, and pointing to the reason for the high grade of immunity enjoyed by these people. Eskimo diet has been discussed in Chapter 3. It becomes important to relate data that sheds light on the habits, manner of life, and physical condition of the primitive, isolated Eskimo of a former day.

Doctors who accompanied expeditions to the Arctic discovered a high level of health among the Eskimos. The more isolated Eskimos were healthier than those who had extensive contact with traders and missionaries. To illuminate this point I can do no better than quote some of the authorities cited in Chapter 3.

Dr. William A. Thomas of the Macmillan Arctic Expedition of 1926 wrote: "Eskimos live on an exclusively meat and fish diet, all eaten usually, and preferably, raw. These people were examined for evidence of renal and vascular disease. The results show conclusively that there was no unusual prevalence of vascular disease or renal disease among 142 adults. The people lead a life of great physical activity. They remain for hours and days in their kayaks, often traveling 24 and 36 hours continuously without rest or food. They frequently alternate between feast and famine. There can, I believe, be no other conclusion than that, under their conditions of life, an exclusively carnivorous diet does not predispose to renal and vascular disease." The average blood pressure of these 142 adults, aged between 40 and 60, was 129 systolic and 76 diastolic. Systolic measures the strength of the heart beat. Diastolic blood pressure is an index of the resistance of the arteries. When the arteries are partially clogged, the resistance to bloodflow (blood pressure) is increased, which in turn requires the heart to pump harder. Although they were not completely isolated from civilization, they had a high measure of good health.

Dr. Thomas contrasts the excellent health of the Eskimos of northern Greenland who have been encouraged by the Danish government to retain their primitive ways, with the poor health of Labrador Eskimos across the Atlantic. These people had been in contact for years with Moravian missions and the Hudson Bay Company. Unfortunately, the Labrador people have abandoned their primitive methods of living. Wood is abundant, so they cook their meat. A distressing situation has developed with the appearance of a number of diseases. In adults there is the rheumatic pain, stiffness of joints, and fatigue so well recognized by the old whalers and explorers as their particular scourge.

Dr. Peter Heinbecker was a member of the Canadian Arctic Expedition of 1931. His tests showed that the "Eskimos had a remarkable power to oxidize fats completely as evidenced by the small amount of acetone excreted in the urine in fasting." Acetone (ketone) bodies in urine indicate ketosis, a state of toxicity that may be induced by a high-fat diet. Dr. Heinbecker seemed surprised by his findings, in view of the quantity of fat consumed.

Dr. I.M. Rabinowitch of the Department of Metabolism, Montreal General Hospital, was with the Canadian Eastern Arctic Patrol in 1925, on the ship R.M.S. Nasopie. He visited Eskimo settlements near Hudson Bay at various distances from trading posts. He took note of evidences of contact with civilization at the various camps, including the introduction of flour. Disease was found to prevail in camps where the inhabitants had given up their primitive diet and substituted a damaged diet. In the more northern camps, where contact with traders was infrequent and where the original diet was used, there was no evidence of arteriosclerosis. In the areas farther south, where the natives adopted some of the ways of the white man, the doctor found that "arteriosclerosis was common, as shown by thickened radial and tortuous temporal vessels," and elevated blood pressure.

Dr. Rabinowitch also made tests on the urine and blood plasma of 34 Eskimos. He found the average chloride blood values higher than for civilized people, while the urine chloride content was extremely low. It is not surprising to find little chloride in the urine because the original Eskimos abhorred adding salt (sodium chloride) to food. When an infrequent visitor gave them some salt as a gift, they would save it and pass it along to the next white man showing up. However, the high chloride level in blood is something very special. The Eskimo, using no salt, has more chloride in the blood than the white man who eats table salt freely. Intact minerals "grown" into raw food speak well for better health, as opposed to isolated "pure" minerals which are randomly added to foods and drugs in civilized societies. Official chemistry, take notice. None of the urines examined by Dr. Rabinowitch contained sugar or acetone. The absence of acetone means that the Eskimo has an unusual ability to utilize fat. Perhaps this can be credited to the lipase the Eskimo eats as a part of the fat in his raw diet.

For about seven years, Dr. J.A. Urquhart carried on a medical practice in the Northwest Territory of Canada, an area of 90,000 square miles. Over this region was scattered a population of 4,000 Eskimos and Indians. The area was visited by dog team, boat, and plane. "The diet of the Eskimos is remarkable for its very high proportion of fat and its almost complete lack of carbohydrate. It consists almost entirely of fat and protein, from caribou, bear, seal, whale, fish, and the fat and blubber of seals and whales," Dr. Urquhart wrote in the *Canadian Medical Association Journal* in 1935. He had not seen a single case of malignancy in either Eskimo or Indian. He analyzed several thousand urine specimens, testing mainly for diabetes and kidney disease.

At first thought, in spite of the evidence, we may be tempted to entertain a vague doubt that lipase has anything to do with the immunity of primitive Eskimos from assault by cholesterol. We may wish to ascribe this immunity to the rigorous frigid climate to which the Eskimo is exposed. But authorities such as V. Stefansson and D.B. MacMillan who have lived with the Eskimos for extended periods agree that permanent Eskimo dwellings were kept at tropical temperatures of 80 to 90° F, or even higher on occasion, by the constant burning of seal-oil lamps. Both the Eskimos and white men living in these domiciles were forced to strip to the waist for many hours due to copious perspiration, which was replenished by continuous drinking of water from melted snow. Some authorities thought that this neutralized possible strain of some of the organ systems of the human body from a heavy intake of meat. When exposed to outside temperatures during work or travel, the Eskimos were efficiently insulated by fur garments, effectively canceling the effect of the frigid weather.

The authorities agreed that the high intake of calories, combined with proper clothing, made the Eskimo comfortable at all times. If the raw diet of Eskimos has had nothing to do with their high standards of health and immunity to disease, how can we explain the poor health and presence of numerous diseases in Eskimos living under identical conditions of climate, but who live near white communities and use a diet more or less extensively cooked?

LIPASE AND DIGESTION

Lipase may benefit us the most when it is allowed to work in successive stages. Whereas pancreatic lipase works high in the alkaline range of the pH scale, lipases in food fats operate more in the acid range (lower in the pH scale). If the fat in food is exposed only to pancreatic lipase, it does not experience the sequence of substrate changes it would undergo had it first been worked on by a food lipase in the cardiac portion of the stomach. It is impossible to rule out the possibility that when enzymes with diverse optimal pH characteristics work on substrates in successive stages, a favorable quality may thereby be imprinted on the resulting products, and be manifested in their future metabolism. The intercourse between fat and its own food lipase takes place every day in the upper part of the digestive tracts of billions of animals. I have called this region the food-enzyme stomach. The very fact that we humans consume cooked food that divorces fat from its lipase, and hinders food enzyme digestion, may actually be the crucial circumstance that breeds mischief into cholesterol. Research costs money, and if we want final proof badly enough it must be paid for. Research might show us how we could take lipase in capsules and end our cholesterol worries.

ENZYME CHANGES IN AGING
AND ARTERIAL DISEASE

Has science learned how many enzymes are kept busy looking after the arteries, and how they are getting along? The scientific periodical literature has been reporting for some years that metabolic enzymes stationed at the arteries are having a difficult time keeping things in order. First of all we may examine whether the digestive enzymes maintain their status with the passage of time. Meyer, Golden, Steiner, and Necheles (1937) reported that a group of 12 subjects, with an average age of 25 years, had a salivary amylase content about 30 times higher than a group of 27 subjects with an average age of 81 years. Meyer, Spier, and Neuwelt (1940) tested pepsin and the pancreatic enzymes of a group of 32 human subjects between 12 and 60 years of age, and a group between 60 and 96 years of age. The younger group had 4 times more pepsin and trypsin than the older, while the lipase was only slightly diminished in the older people. Drs. Becker, Meyer, and Necheles found that in older persons the amount of lipase was relatively low in pancreatic juice, and was accompanied by slow fat absorption from the intestine. These findings lead to the speculation that in hardening of the arteries, some fat may be absorbed in the unhydrolyzed (undigested or partially digested) state. The experimenters fed lipase to both young and old subjects and demonstrated that there was definite improvement in fat utilization. There are many other reports pointing in the direction that older arteries have been suffering for years, trying to get along with too few enzymes. Bad arteries hurt the heart two ways. Clogged arteries in the heart muscle stop feeding it, causing a heart attack. Hard arteries elsewhere make the heart work too hard and the result is high blood pressure and the dangers of a possible stroke.

In a 1942 investigation, Meyer, Sorter, and Necheles checked blood serum enzymes. At an average age of 77, the serum lipase was 1.50 units, while at an average of 27, serum lipase was 2.04 units. The serum amylase level, however, was no different. Bernhard (1951) tested serum lipase in normal, hypertensive, and arteriosclerotic male and female adult humans and found it subnormal in hypertensive and arteriosclerotic males, but normal in the females. Malkov (1964) discovered "that the lipoprotein lipase activities of the aortas of old rats and rabbits were significantly lower than those of young animals of the same species respectively." Rats, which are resistant to the development of atherosclerosis, manifested about twice the aortic lipoprotein lipase activities that rabbits did, the latter animals being notorious for the ease with which they develop the disease.

Dr. J.E. Kirk published an ambitious compendium of global literature on enzymes of the arterial wall. The tabulations in his 1969 book, Enzymes of the Arterial Wall, covered 27,200 assays on 98 different enzymes. The values are presented in 278 tables. In one table, representing 131 instances of arteriosclerosis of the aorta and coronary arteries, 49 showed lowered enzyme activity, 18 showed elevated enzyme activity, and 64 showed enzyme activity unchanged. Dr. Kirk stated: "Extended enzyme studies will undoubtedly provide an opportunity for identification of some of the local metabolic factors associated with the pathogenesis of arteriosclerosis. The efforts presently being made in enzyme research make us hopeful about the final outcome."

Zempleny (1974) wrote that the activity of most enzymes shows significant alterations in atherosclerotic arteries, but that investigation of advanced lesions does not answer the question whether such activity changes precede atherosclerosis, or result from the development of the disease. From this I can draw the conclusion that in arterial disease, enzyme activities in the arteries are indeed merely a strained reactive mechanism—makeshift defensive measures. An evaluation of the evidence presented in this treatise justifies the opinion that the underlying cause of atherosclerosis reverts to maldigestion of fat in the digestive tract, and absorption of defective fatty products.

SOME LIPASE IN BLOOD COMES FROM RAW FOOD

Horvath (1926), a physiologist, wrote: "The presence of lipase in numerous foods of vegetable and animal origin led us to suppose their lipases might also be one of the sources of lipase supply in living organisms." To test this theory, it was necessary to determine if enzymes could in fact be absorbed by the membranes of the small intestine, a controversial subject. Accordingly, raw soybeans with their lipase, were fed to rabbits and the serum lipase level became elevated. Measures were then employed to insure that the soybean lipase had actually been absorbed, and that the serum lipase level did not coincidentally rise from stimulation of endogenous lipase by the fat of soybean. Another startling report comes by way of a German medical journal, claiming that the lipase content of adipose tissue from cases of human obesity, and from lipomas, was found to be less than normal.

EATING REFINED VEGETABLE FAT
CAUSED CANCER AMONG 423 MEN

There is a worldwide attempt to control cardiovascular disease by limiting or excluding the intake of animal fat in all forms, including dairy products. As substitutes, highly purified vegetable oils are frequently recommended. These are crystal-clear products, pure fat, with the same blemished nutritional pedigree that pure, white table sugar has had to endure these many years. Any isolated, purified, skeletonized food material must be expected to have adverse, far-reaching effects on the health of living organisms. This can be predicted by the history of human nutrition.

It need not be unduly surprising to read the report entitled, "Incidence of Cancer in Men on Diet High in Polyunsaturated Fat." Universities and the Veterans Administration in the Los Angeles area collaborated in a clinical trial extending over 8 years to test the efficacy of a diet in which vegetable oils were substituted for saturated fat. The test involved 846 men living in government hospitals. Half of them were kept on a diet with purified, unsaturated fats, while the other half ate a regular diet with ordinary fats, including butter. Those eating unsaturated purified fat had lower blood cholesterol levels and fewer deaths from cardiovascular diseases, 48 versus 70. An unexpected finding after the 8 years of the diet was that of the 423 subjects eating the purified fat there were 31 cancer deaths, while in the 423 eating some animal fat there were only 17 deaths from cancer. In a press conference in 1971, the architects of the program, Drs. M.L. Pearce and S. Dayton, of the University of California, issued a warning to go slow both on cholesterol and purified oils.

EFFORTS IN ENZYME RESEARCH

Before food enzymes can come into their own in monitoring the control of human disease, money is needed to push modern research in the whole subject of enzyme nutrition. For example, the optimum dosage of lipase extract must be experimentally determined. It has been found that a certain type of dehydrated lipase powder works longer in the first part of the stomach. Persons with artery disease and its elevated blood pressure could swallow the lipase capsules to fight cholesterol. How many and how often would have to be determined, however. Only the clinics in hospitals and other institutions could bring together enough patients to do justice to such a program in a reasonable time. Another experimental approach is to develop atherosclerosis in laboratory animals and then test out the lipase extract on them, to see what it does to their blood pressure and cholesterol deposits. What is needed is more funding for this crucial research.

Appendix A

Enzymes, Soil, and Agriculture

Scientists are now measuring the value of a soil by the amount of enzymes it contains. These enzyme values have a direct relationship to the quality of our nutrition and health. Some technicians prefer to test for the enzyme dehydrogenase. Others look for the enzymes amylase, urease, asparaginase, cellulase, invertase, phosphatase, phytase, protease, saccharase, or xylanase. It is known that the operation of microorganisms in the soil is very important to the growth of plants. The world is commencing to awaken to the importance of enzymes in the life of the soil—the biological activity of the soil. A plant, like an animal, needs enzymes to prosper. While the enzymes present in soil bacteria help to supply this need, good soil also contains free enzymes. While the enzymes present in soil are under consideration, mention may be made of the popularity of the mud bath in the treatment of disease in Europe. In 1956, F.M. Bilyans'kii of the Russian Institute of Biochemistry stated that the curative property of muds has been commonly ascribed to the presence of the enzyme catalase.

In connection with the enrichment of the soil, the enzyme contributions of earthworms should not be ignored. Charles Darwin realized the part worms have played in building soil and wrote a treatise on the subject. In the act of burrowing through the earth, worms engulf the soil and extract usable materials as food. After passing through the length of the worm, the remainder is expelled in the form of casts which contain a valuable contribution of worm enzyme excretions. Worms, like all other animals, continually take in enzymes and eliminate them in their excretions, giving the soil an endowment of free enzymes. Soil rich in worm casts is sought after by some horticulturists for the cultivation of favored plants. It makes high-grade plant food.

Worms not only add enzymes to the soil but also loosen it, permitting water and air deeper access. Years ago I witnessed the proficiency of the common night crawler, *lumbricus terrestris*, as recycling specialists. In the autumn we would store fallen leaves in barrels. The following spring a shallow layer of leaves was strewn over the surface of my worm pit. The worms would come up at night and devour the leaves, leaving the surface barren in several days, when more leaves would be spread. Although the worm pit was small, all of the leaves from the previous autumn were cleaned up in this way. Later, the soil in the pit was used in the garden.

Synthetic, enzymeless fertilizers were developed only about 50 or 60 years ago. For thousands of years before that, farmers had been using enzyme-rich manure. And for untold millions of years before farming began, soil had been receiving the fresh urine and feces from countless numbers of animals and birds. Vast herds comprising millions of animals roamed the land. Enormous flocks of birds blotted out the sky. And all of these creatures dropped their enzyme-laden urine and feces on the soil to fertilize it according to the plan of nature. When these millions finally died, their bodies dropped to the ground, the soil inheriting a good share of their enzymes. Any physiologist will confirm that these animal and human waste products are rich in enzymes resulting from normal wear and tear. Although they are not good enough to retain in an organism's body, they have proven their worth for millenniums.

Scientists from many countries have discovered free enzymes (as opposed to those present in bacteria) in the soil. For thousands of years farmers have been fertilizing their fields with manure. Manure, an enzyme fertilizer, is an excelleent source of free enzymes because it is made of urine, feces, and straw. Of course, when manure accumulates in piles for months and is rained on repeatedly, some of the enzymes are washed away and wasted. What right have we to deny these enzymes to the soil and spread synthetic, enzymeless fertilizer—along with the fiction that it is just as good?

The enzymeless fertilizer substitutes weaken vegetables and other plant foods, building up a hidden preclinical entity, a state of "disease" that is a prelude to disease. Poisonous sprays do not cure the lowered vitality responsble for this state—instead they kill the plant predators and thereby prevent the vegetables, grains, and fruits from being destroyed by real disease. Every farmer knows his crops are so lowered in vitality that they would be ruined in the fields if their predators were not killed by poison. Modern crops cannot stand on their own feet without the aid of poison. Just think about the fact that we all eat this nearly diseased food! Livestock also eat it and pass on the predisposition to disease to us when we consume meat, fowl, and dairy products. The weak state of vegetable and animal food can be a factor in many serious human diseases.

"The survival of the fittest" is a law that prevailed in nature for millions of years. The weakest plants and animals perished; the most vigorous and healthiest survived to continue the species. Living up to modern doctrines, we have recently developed respect for and stopped maligning such predators as the lion, wolf, and eagle, and now protect them as part of nature's scheme. But we have been taught to believe in a double standard which ordains death for plant predators. We have become conditioned to think of these visible and microscopic health officers of the soil, not as nature's predators, responsible for destroying weak plants and keeping up a high standard of health in the vegetable kingdom, but as pests, to be killed any way possible. Students are led to believe nature made a mistake. The law of predation was more or less allowed to apply to both the animal and vegetable kingdoms until some three score years ago when synthetic, artificial, enzymeless fertilizers made their appearance. All at once plants could not hold their own and began to be attacked and afflicted with numerous ailments which had been no real problem when enzyme fertilizers were employed. The fact that powerful poisons must be universally used by farmers to enable crops to survive, proves that the foods we eat are really miserable weaklings, unable to measure up to the standard demanded by "the survival of the fittest." We ignore nature's law and use poisons to destroy plant predators and seem to feel no guilt at all in promoting the survival of the "unfittest."

Appendix B
Research Contribution

By Maynard Murray, M.D.

Dr. Murray was Medical Director of Sunland, a
large Florida state institution. The author of the
book *Sea Energy Agriculture* and of many contributions to the scientific periodical literature, he
was also an eye, ear, nose, and throat specialist.

INTRODUCTION

During the course of a conversation with Dr. Murray, he casually
mentioned some highly illuminating research findings which have a
profound bearing on health and disease. I asked him in which journals
he had reported details about these findings and was shocked to learn
this valuable research had never been reported. I pleaded with Dr.
Murray that the world is starving for this kind of information, where-
upon he graciously agreed to assemble and write up the data and
have it published in this book.

The first valuable report relates the treatment of 5 patients afflicted
with epilepsy, by oral administration of plant protease, amylase, and
lipase enzymes in capsules, and the determination of the effect on
their blood magnesium levels and brain waves.

In the second report Dr. Murray relates participating in anatomical
dissection of whales and seals and unearthing the astounding and
challenging revelation that their arteries were healthy, free from
cholesterol, in spite of the fact that their harsh environment requires
consumption of fat wihout restraint. We have to answer the important
question why these warm-blooded animals can eat large amounts of
fat with impunity, while we are punished with atherosclerosis. Whales
and seals need a heavy layer of insulating fat under the skin to keep

warm and should be prime candidates for atherosclerosis, but they have none. A summary of the two reports follows, in Dr. Murray's own words.

ENZYME THERAPY IN EPILEPSY

Enclosed you will find a list of 5 patients, all of whom had low blood magnesium levels. They had been treated for this condition without effect for at least 5 years. In 3 months on the enzymes all of their blood magnesium levels came up to normal. You will also see the results of EEG's (brain waves) run on these same 5 patients; 4 out of 5 showed change for the better in the brain wave. This, of course, is a very small group, but due to the percentage improvement, the therapy should be given to a much larger number. The dosage of magnesium gluconate was one gram, 4 times a day. Enzymes were given 3 times a day after meals, 2 capsules each time. I hope this information will be of help and interest to you.

EFFECTS OF ENZYME THERAPY

Name of Patient	Blood Magnesium Levels (in millequivalents/liter)		EEG Date	EEG Date
	Oct. 18, 1979	Jan. 14, 1980		
Brenda C.	1.25 mEq/l	1.42 mEq/l	3-25-77	1-11-80
Sandra H.	1.18 mEq/l	1.33 mEq/l	5-31-79	1-10-80
William H.	1.30 mEq/l	1.50 mEq/l	10-29-76	1-10-80
James M.	1.26 mEq/l	1.53 mEq/l	5-22-79	1-10-80
Joan McC.	1.24 mEq/l	1.35 mEQ/l	10-21-77	1-11-80

INTERPRETATION OF EEG RESULTS

Brenda C.: Relatively unchanged. The present function is better than that seen in 1977.

Sandra H.: This does represent some improvement since the previous record.

William H.: The true seizure activity noted previously is not seen in this record and this does represent a significant change.

James M.: The general impression is that it is a little improvement over the previous record but the change is not great.

Joan McC.: There has been very little change since the last record.

FAT IN WHALES AND SEALS

Within the years 1942–1945, under the auspices of Archer, Daniels, Midland Company of Chicago, between 900–1000 sperm whales were dissected in Peru. The only pathology sought in these animals involved malignancies, arteriosclerosis, and arthritis. None of these were found. We also measured the size of the thymus gland which persisted in these animals; weight 80 to 100 pounds in the slaughtered carcass. While microscopic sections of these glands were not numerous, however, the tissue examined showed them to be active and not replaced by fat or fibrous tissue. The coronary arteries microscopically did not show any atherosclerosis; neither did the aortas. There was approximately 8 inches of saturated subcutaneous fat in whales, yet no hardening of the arteries.

Off of the Aleutian Islands of Alaska, around 3,000 seals were dissected after being slaughtered for their fur. No malignant tumors were found, and there was no pathology in their arteries and joints. We dissected about 30 small Harp Seals which were slaughtered on ice floes off the eastern coast of Canada. These animals also showed no pathology of the kinds mentioned above.

Maynard Murray, M.D.

About Dr. Howell

Dr. Edward Howell was born in Chicago in 1898. He holds a limited medical license from the State of Illinois. (The holder of a limited practice license must pass the same Board Examination as a medical doctor. Only materia medica, obstetrics, and surgery are excluded.)

In 1924, after obtaining his license, Dr. Howell joined the staff of the Lindlahr Sanitarium in Illinois, where he remained until 1930. He then established a private practice for the treatment of advanced illness utilizing nutritional and physical therapies. For the next 40 years until his retirement he spent three days each week with patients, while the balance of his time was devoted to various kinds of research.

Dr. Howell is the true pioneer in his field, having been the first researcher to recognize and delineate the importance of the enzymes in food to human nutrition. In 1946 he wrote *The Status of Food Enzymes in Digestion and Metabolism*, which has recently been reprinted. He then took more than 20 years to complete *Enzyme Nutrition*, of which this book is a published abridgment. The original is approximately 700 pages long and contains over 700 references to the world's scientific literature.

Dr. Howell, now eighty-seven, is presently living in Southwest Florida where he serves as Research Director for the Food Enzyme Research Foundation and continues his writing and research.

Index

Adams, C.W. et al., 147
Agriculture, enzyme
time-honored; modern farming
enzymeless, 157–159
for millenniums nature manured
soil by animal excretions, 157–158
animal excretions rich in
enzymes, 23, 27, 33, 126, 157
farmers used enzyme manure fertilizer thousands of years, 157–158
synthetic enzymeless fertilizer made
food diseased, 158
animal predators kill the weak—
keep species vigorous, 159
"insect pests" are plant predators—
soil's health officers, 159
plant predators destroy diseased
food—protect humans, 159
enzymeless fertilizers need poison
to grow even bad food, 157–159
poisons destroy plant predators—
result, diseased food, 159
we use a dubious double standard—
protect animal predators, 159
kill plant predators and eat diseased
"near" food, 159
Allergies
modern allergy concept developed
in early 1920s, 140
old concept goes back many years
and applies only to raw food,
139–144
food enzymes purge evil substrates
—itching eruptions exit, 141

food and body enzymes cleanse
body by bowel and lung
discharges, 139–144
stopping these constructive efforts
may be contraindicated, 139–144
to test a raw food allergy, find least
amount of causative food, 142
eat half of this amount daily, 142
after a reasonable period return to
the original amount, 142
if no symptoms appear build up
intake slowly, 142
use of supplemental enzymes in
allergies, 143–144
Andrus, S.B., 78–79
Arky, R., 90
Arteries. *See also* Calories; Cholesterol;
Eskimos; Obesity.
cholesterol and faulty fat digestion
and metabolism, 145–156
optimal metabolism uses different
enzymes to digest fat, 145–146, 153
fat not properly predigested may not
be well metabolized, 147–149
lipase is present in all raw foods
containing fat, 147
in human obesity and fatty tumors,
lipase subnormal, 147
human artery enzymes progressively
weaker after middle age, 154–155
artery enzymes become weaker in
atherosclerosis, 154–155
in dogs with atherosclerosis,
associated blood enzymes low, 147